Christa Nehls

Living beyond Pain
Your journey to a fulfilled life

A guide to overcome pain based
on the L.I.S.A.-Method ®

May 2002 / August 2008 /
November 2012 / Summer 2013

**Volume 2 of the series
„Actions speak louder than words"**

© Copyright: Publishing House Menschin

All rights reserved.
Copyright © 2013 by
Publishing House Menschin Christa Nehls
68165 Mannheim, Germany
Translation: Christin Greif
Design: selicht, Langenargen

All rights reserved. No part of this publication may be translated, reproduced, stored in a retrieval system, or transmitted, in any form or by any means, electronic, mechanical, photocopying, recording or otherwise, without the prior permission of the publisher.

Printed in Germany.

www.menschin.com

ISBN 978-3-944126-04-3

Dedicated to my Dad,
who always believed in me,
who taught me
never to give up,
ever to stand up tall, keep going on,
and question
whether the road I took
was the right one, and if not,
to shift to the right course.

R.I.P. September 2012

Thanks

Dream it.
Do it.
And you will make it.

Sergio Bambaren

I owe gratitude to many people,
to those who encouraged me and gave me the strength to keep on working on this project, but above all to those who believe in me. Thanks to the many patients who trusted me over and over again, who gave me the strength throughout the course of my work and effort to effectuate better medical care for pain patients.

Christa Nehls

Table of Contents

Preface **13**

Part I – My Story under the reign of pain **15**

The following weeks 21

Finally, a helping hand 23

A car seat and its consequences 37

Treatment or rehabilitation…? 41

A year later 47

Part II – Words of Contemplation **51**

Words from the Depths of my Exhaustion 55

Words breaking free from me 59

Conciliating words: Pain therapist and Pain patient 61

Part III – From pain patient to pain person. Become your own coach. **65**

A word on implementation 67

It's my playground 71

Relaxation 73

Back to me – Beginning and End 75

Is it okay to be selfish? 77

The 8 golden seconds 81

Gathering and assessing information...85

Information – and what now?...89

Pain, Friends and Loneliness 93

Yet another facet of life-quality 95

Pain Patients' "Actions" really "speaking louder than words".....99

I repeat and recapitulate..103

Working Hand in Hand...105

Part IV – Case Studies   **107**

An Introduction to Case Ctudies 109

Hell with every touch..111

My life isn't worthwhile 113

Words are my last anchor...115

Can't keep up anymore..117

Hitting a dead end..119

Not forgiving me...121

Pain, don't leave me all alone!...123

Did you buy that 125

No one listens to me..129

Summary 131

Part V – Self-help Groups   **135**

Self-help Groups..137

A few words about the internet and its utilization 141

International Links..143

Stories for Encouragement and Relaxation 145

Part VI – Appendix   **149**

Questionnaire about pain 151

Closing Word 157

Preface

This book is to encourage pain patients, yes; this is exactly what you are holding in your hands: a book to support you and give you courage,

- Courage, to accept your pain.
- Courage, to cope with your pain.
- Courage, to be yourself throughout your pain.
- Courage, to keep your pain under control.
- Courage, to lead a self-determined life.

In the first part of this book, I will tell you my own story with pain. I wish to pass some courage on to other pain suffering people and to assure them, that everything will be alright. Not even I have a miraculous cure to offer, but only courage, much courage and patience. Whatever may come, stay strong, hang on and do not give up! Which reminds me of a song from the eighties:

„I beg your pardon, I never promised you a rose garden, along with the sunshine, there's gotta be a little rain sometime..." performed by Lynn Anderson.

In this book, I will tell you more about the way to regain control of your life, the way to earn your doctor's esteem and to gradually become the master of your own life again. Words are easy, I know. Actions speak louder than words, after all. It is all up to you. So take action, take over the reins and fashion the life you want to live. All you have is a single chance, a single life. So stay strong! Arm yourself with the following motto:

We never know for sure,
if anything will get better,
if we make a change.
Yet we know for sure,
we have got to make a change,
if we want anything to get better.

Are you having a weird feeling in your gut? That is part of it.

Do you remember yourself as a lonely child in the woods, surrounded with rustling, whispering sounds and that big scary arm (just a branch) trying to get you? Everything seemed strange and frightening then. You will always be haunted with such feelings when you strike out on a new path, your escort will be insecurity and fear. You might be thinking now: this does not sound good. But I tell you it sounds actually very good, because every time you will find yourself in this state of mind, you will know you hit a new path.

May 2002, February 2005, August 2008, August 2013

Part I – My Story under the reign of pain

My unwelcome guest...

... it appeared all of a sudden, uninvited, it came and annoyed. A pain in every aspect of my life, it destroyed the life I used to lead, the life I drifted along day in day out.
I had turned 40 about seven months earlier and had thus reached the midlife crisis. A crisis I had neither the will nor the time for. It was so important to live my life, one day after the other, but this unbidden guest simply showed me how different life really is... he, my pain, I suddenly should, or rather had, to share my life with.

The beginnings

Everything began on a beautiful summer morning, on the 20th of June 1997 about 10:30 o'clock as I tried to stand up from my office chair... in vain! I tried again and again, but all I scored was a succession of failures. Finally I gave up trying and thought to myself: only a short time ago, about one or two hours ago, I could still stand up, but it was not necessary at the time. Now, I want to stand up! The longer I thought about it, the stronger grew the urge to be able to stand. Panic rushed through my head, through my entire body. Every inch of me wanted to stand up...but couldn't. So I leaned with my hands on my desk very slowly, with the tips of my fingers pointing inwards opposing each other, the handballs facing outwards, pulling up my weight with all my power, I somehow painfully managed to raise my body and prop it against my hands.

I finally managed to speak, so I told my colleague that "I am having pain in the back". And he answered: "Oh, just ignore it; it's probably not as bad as you think".
Some time passed off and we went over to another building for lunch. The thought I had managed to walk flashed through my head. After lunch we returned to the office, I sat down and worked at my computer...after a while, I decided I had to get some water to quench my thirst. But I couldn't get off the chair. The damn terror began all over again.

My colleague – being apparently more attentive this time – said I should „go home, it seems to be pretty bad." and said he couldn't "bear seeing me like this". So I thought "shut up, you're bugging me". Walking relieves the pain and I had already brought some water to drink.

Nevertheless, I went pretty scared home. It was a Friday afternoon, in the early summer 1997. At this time in Germany, doctors were already off duty.

I thought „It's not so bad", „this all will be over soon" and so came Saturday. We received an invitation and I kept thinking "it's not so bad", so we agreed to go. Sunday went by...without any improvement. I clung to the thought "it's not so bad", this is nothing but mere pain. Monday, the doctor would surely know where the pain is exactly emanating from and prescribe some medication and all of this will be history".
The family doctor examined me on Monday and shortly diagnosed it was the "sciatic nerve", I was given an injection (the usual remedy) but the pain was not appeased. I was told "in a couple of hours the pain will fade away and on Thursday you can go back to work".

But, on Thursday, I couldn't go to work because the pain had grown even stronger. I couldn't even remain seated in the waiting room, so I paced up and down the hallway of the doctor's office.
My pacing irritated the other waiting patients, sometimes later I was called into a treatment room. Again I was given an injection, and again it was useless. A week later, the pain grew even worse, so I was given yet another injection along with a referral to the orthopedic.

Now, I was categorized. I have a problem in the locomotor system.

The pain tormented me with sleepless nights. In the meantime I could only – if at all – walk, sit, lie, stand, drive, sleep or eat under the impact of pain that became an inseparable, yet unbidden companion.
Each movement was torture; life was a series of continuous sufferings. Why me? What have I done to deserve this hell? I hated the pain. Leave me alone, go away, I never asked for you, so beat it!!!
Great, I had to bear waiting in crowded waiting rooms, with pain pushing me to tears...tears of despair...of distress...of feelings even I could not describe...

And there I was waiting for my rescuer, the orthopedic. I only managed for a few minutes to stay seated before I started pacing about in a waiting room opened to the office's hallway and reception desk. The other waiting patients were irritated by my pacing here too – Oh, how I wished I didn't have to bear all that pain – I could even understand their irritation.
I referred to the doctor's assistants and asked whether it may be possible to let me in ahead of time, but everyone around could hear us talking, so I wasn't allowed to jump the queue. And the

waiting lasted… and lasted. It lasted two long hours, or three, or… forever and I felt rather dead than alive.

Finally I was X-rayed. Every possible reflex of body had to be tested, and the doctor asked a long series of questions. Finally he pressed a pack of Ibuprofen into my hands and sent me home. „So, this should relief your pain pretty fast. We could also recourse to a little bit of physiotherapy, using cervical traction or stretching, I have the necessary machine right here."
But I always felt dizzy after stretching, "so we should drop that, anyway I couldn't get to the bottom of your problem. Are you sure you want more painkillers?"
And so my pain and I were given a new nickname: "The pretender". I never felt so miserable in my entire life. "Pretender" the word flashed through my mind, I was bruised into an emotional rollercoaster, "pretender", "stop pretending".

The following weeks

I tried to get back to work, and managed to hang on in there for three hours before I hobbled through the building back to the car and drove home, feeling miserable as sin, useless, dispensable and alone with my pain, the caring words of my boss still echoing in the back of my mind: "Just do the necessary and go home, I cannot bear seeing you having all this pain".

The family doctor was at a loss as to what to do, thought about the neurologist and reckoned, that if all else fails, we could still recourse to the pain clinic next town. Then we ruled out the last option; the neurologist seemed to be the better solution.

Obviously, I kept trying to keep everything under control at home and in the garden. The next time I went shopping at the garden center, I found a swing with two seats that I just couldn't resist buying. The vendor managed it, with quite some effort though, to disassemble the swing and maneuver it into my car. This swing saved me all through the summer. It became my refuge, my place of peace. And so it still is till this day, every time I am lost in distress or feeling about to suffocate.

This swing is my anchor. But still, after all those beats and blows, I was more and more feeling devastated, trampled underfoot, wandering in the undergrounds of misery. Some of my friends began to feel annoyed as I told them on the phone that "I can't make it to your house with all this pain", or that "the pain is still same old same old…", and soon they stopped calling. I didn't call them anymore either; I was too busy suffering.

My strengths wore ever thinner. My partner tried, but couldn't really understand what was wrong with me. He knew I was not doing well, but couldn't cope with the situation. How should he anyway, if not even I managed to. The atmosphere at home kept growing ever gloomier. I was alone! This realization raided my heart and mind like an avalanche. Nobody helped, nobody could. The avalanche in my heart suffocated the last bits of strength left in me; I was completely drained of all my power.

My neighbor was my sole support. I sometimes used to actually lie in wait for her to come back home. She spoke to me, encouraged me…she kept me going on, at least until the next day. There were two more people taking care of me: one of them was a friend living quite far away from me – in Cologne, half the world away – who called me every Monday afternoon. Her words were some help and comfort. She was at the same my colleague, and that's how I at least got to know some of what was going on in the office and in the company. None of my other colleagues cared. Once, my boss called to ask whether I would like to come back to the office and distract myself a little, which probably would help me get well faster. And a client even called me every now and then; he encouraged me and told me how much he admires my endurance.

Finally, a helping hand

The neurologist examined my reflexes, all of them were alright. He also happened to be a psychotherapist. So he suggested a few other major tests and examinations such as CAT scanning and MRI. The neurologist lived about 22 miles away in a large city named Mannheim. Not far from himyou was a joint practice for radiology. As I trudged myself there to my appointment, I was CAT scanned right away. "You can barely stand and you come from far away. We just happen to have some free time, follow me please. It is better for you to wait for five minutes here than having to come over for a second appointment." The lady was nice to me... which moved me to tears, again. I was CAT scanned with much care. This time it came out that a lumbar vertebra has so strongly rotated, that it was pinching the nerves going through one of the two vertebral canals.

I underwent an MRI a couple of days later. Oh! How I hated the tight tube, I feared the constriction; I was having so much pain and couldn't lie straight on my back. The neurologist gave me a tranquilizer to take before the beginning of the examination in the scanning tube. But then I couldn't drive, so I asked my partner to drive me. He was irritated. He just didn't understand the situation. He didn't like driving me to the MRI; to him, it was an unbearable burden; he couldn't understand my fear of the tube, but above all, my fear...

I lied in the tube. A doctor stayed by my side all the time with his hand on my foot so that I could feel his presence. He kept talking to me; as much as the noise of the MRI allowed him to. He asked me every now and then if I could still remain laid down, then another thicker and softer pillow was put beneath me replacing the hard standard pillow. Even my partner stayed close to the scanning tube, bearing the noise in spite of everything.

Both MRI and CAT scan lead to the same result: the vertebrae S1/L5 had slipped against each other…mine were moving like pearls on a string. One of the spinal canals through which the nerves exit the spinal column was already completely blocked under the impact of the pressure.

With this diagnosis I went back to the family doctor. She decided I need physiotherapy, soon after that she went on vacation. Her superior treated me as if I were an impostor and was even rude to me. That was really the last thing I needed! He was not even able to adequately evaluate the CAT and MRI images, "oh, we are quite familiar with this stuff, it is our day-to-day work here" he said. What an absolute nonsense!

Physiotherapy didn't help…

The health insurance company was really supportive back then. The person responsible for my case took wholeheartedly care of me without hesitation. Sickness benefits, no problem! I received 100% compensation for 26 weeks from the part of the employer without any problem. They even contacted my employer themselves and settled everything. The insurance company provided me moreover with an application form for gradual re-integration in the employment market. Now that I knew what was wrong with me, on the physical level, I wanted to work again. It was early August 1997.

I couldn't bear staying home anymore. Not even the public library had any more interesting books for me in store, neither could the book shop offer me anything exciting anymore, instead my parents did: "Ayla and the bear clan". I devoured the novel and even cried many passages through. The origins of communication were therein unveiled: sign language. I began ever since to watch the weekly "Seeing, not hearing" show. During that time, I read a pocketbook every day, while my wallet was overburdened with my persistent book-shopping and my back with the long steep stairs to the public library. But I didn't give up. I clung to this tiny pleasure of losing myself in stories, forgetting my pain, hiding from the tormenting pain, or better yet, chasing it out of my mind. It turned out later, that by tending to my pain with rest, I had actually done myself anything else but a favor.

I tried to „re-integrate", but sadly the attempt remained only empty words. I managed to endure two days at the office, only for four hours on each; on the third day I broke out in tears and left after only two hours, thus giving up on the attempt to re-integrate. It was, I think, August 20th , 1997.

I was devastated. Everything seemed vain. I didn't want to live anymore.

But somehow I lived on. Over the following week, I lived through my darkest hours till then. I cried 24 hours through. I had to find my balance on a narrow edge, like the one of a crater, beset by sharp slope walls over and underneath me, walls ending up in a deep black hole, geometrically perfect, like the inside of an inverted pyramid…and battling with infinite fear.
By Tuesday however, I had won the battle and decided to stand up for myself: I wanted to live!

I asked myself over and over again: "what could there be behind a black hole?" My mind slowly began to take over, putting my feelings in leash for a change. On my last job as medical record engineer, I once visited a pain clinic in "Mainz", about twenty years ago. I hoped that clinic still existed, that there would be even more such clinics by now. Wait! The family doctor said something about an outpatient pain clinic, so where's the phonebook. I was struck by the cruel realization: There is no pain clinic in town! Take it easy, breathe! Think! Hospitals do have outpatient clinics…We have two local hospitals; I decided to call one of them. "No, we don't have a pain clinic here", I was told, "but the other hospital does, I'll give you the phone number". Great, there was someone helping without me even asking. All I said was "Thank you", still puzzled though, then I called the number I was just given.

I was immediately connected with the pain clinic, all this happened on Tuesday. I was supposed to drop by on Friday afternoon and bring along any documents I had. Hoppla, there was someone thinking! Something I hadn't seen any more since a quite long time. The time I spent waiting for Friday was damn long, but the promised Friday afternoon came at last. I had trouble getting into the car, I had trouble driving about two and a half miles to the pain clinic of the hospital next town. The rooms were situated right behind the reception, so I got a turn almost immediately.
This was the first time I met people suffering as much as I; whose minds were consumed with pain, as much as mine; whose every move was accompanied with pain, like mine. They comforted me as I was not received on due time saying "this is normal because the staff sometimes has to tend to emergencies. But don't worry, you surely will get help here." I believed them.

There, I met the doctor, the anesthesiologist, the palliative doctor, all in one and the same person; finally after two months of incessant excruciating pain. This doctor dedicated two hours to me. He talked to me, he read every written document carefully through (even though there wasn't so much to read anyway), he examined all the images I brought along. He explained me what those images reveal, he explained me the causes of my pain and their possible origins in my past. He suggested more tests to be conducted by the gynecologist, in order to rule out any further possible causes.
He suggested I should make an EDA (epidural anesthesia), no, he told me, he would give me the EDA on Monday himself (he was absolutely right about that). I shouldn't drive to the hospital by myself, he said. I was confused so he explained his reasons. I finally understood that an analgesic is going to be injected near the spinal canal …I was so afraid. It became clear to me that this was the only way for me to become "treatable". And yet, I was so afraid.

Monday, I went back to the clinic, my sole companions were a strong diarrhea, a still rising fear and the pity of the taxi driver. I got the EDA injection, then the taxi driver picked me up again as I called her, she was the head of the taxi-service company. She drove me home and saw to that I arrive safe and sound to my apartment. That afternoon I felt actually really well. But over night and on the next day, my situation severely deteriorated and I had horrible headaches. The recommended coke, painkillers and much liquid drinking were no help at all against the torments. I just wanted the stabbing pain in my spine to stop. I was so afraid that I didn't even dare to go to the clinic…the pain was just killing me.

At some point in time, anything seems easier to endure than such pain.

On Thursday morning, I underwent an epidural blood patch, on Friday afternoon I was for the first time after 11 weeks free of pain. Now, I could sit down and eat without being tormented. I had spent the night before on a drip in the hospital because of dehydration.

Then I went back home. As of that day, I put my pain therapist on a pedestal. He really succeeded in taking away the pain and gave me forms to help me keep a journal. He referred me to a physiotherapist specialized in the treatment of pain patients.

Now, I was finally really "treatable" and to be helped take action... Being "treatable" means that a doctor could now treat me without me screaming of pain at the slightest movement or touch.

The health insurance expert doctors wanted to see me to check up how sick I really was. The doctors treated me quite kindly as they examined me and verified all the documents I brought along. They decided I should immediately be admitted into a treatment and rehabilitation center. Fighting out a new battle was at hand.

Mid-September I had my first appointment with the physiotherapist. Afterwards, I had three appointments each week, many weeks over. He managed to get at the pain, examined me meticulously before moving to the practical part and so I underwent manual therapy.

Driving over 15 miles before reaching the therapist's office felt like going through hell, I sometimes didn't even know how I got there anymore. He organized a program for me to follow at home. After all, I had much time on my hands because I couldn't work anyway. At that stage, I was unable to do any housework myself, but fortunately, I had engaged a helping hand a year earlier. The physiotherapist got at my pain, he reached and understood me while the painful therapy often pushed me to tears, that officially so-called "manual therapy".

Sometimes, when my mind was not completely paralyzed by pain, I noticed that even my physiotherapist was shocked at the immense pain I suffered at his slightest touch. Yet, we were getting along, slowly, painfully, but steadily.

Step by step, I regained trust in my feet…in my entire body. My physiotherapist encouraged me to go out on walks, alone. Only very short ones for a start, about 50 yards, then 100 yards, then a bit more every day. One day, I was able to report with much pride, I had "managed to walk an entire mile within a good 40 minutes, all by myself", with emphasis of "an entire" and "all by myself". I kept practicing every day, until I managed a few weeks later to walk a mile within just 30 minutes, and a couple of months later, within around 20 minutes. Ever since, I was regularly to be found walking in the old park at the "Rhine" river nearby, most of all on Saturdays and Sundays, on some wonderful summer mornings or even at seven a.m. before the sun was high in the sky.

My confidence grew day by day. I went regularly to the appointments at the outpatient pain clinic, mostly for consultation; I didn't get any more painkillers, except upon my express request, but I didn't need any, I could now manage without them.

In late October I had become very courageous, so I bought myself a ticket for a musical in -"Mannheim"- a big town, about 22 miles away from home, my great joy was mixed with some fear. Sitting there for two hours besides driving to the theater and back was absolute torture for my back. But the show was wonderful, and I had finally dared to take part in social life again. My companions were worried about me, but all I wanted was to enjoy my time. I won back a tiny piece of freedom...I was not enslaved by pain anymore.

Afterwards, I dared a more extreme attempt: I want to take another try on reintegration. It began about the end of October 1997. But this time, I was armed with more knowledge, so I began working two hours a day for two weeks long. Every second week I added a working hour. My physiotherapist expressed his serious concerns, the health insurance company tried to warn me, I shouldn't overstrain myself, my pain therapist supported my request... but my family doctor was clueless.

It worked. Fortunately, the company I worked for had decided to give me a laptop to work on at home, so I could at least read my e-mails. That way, I would not be completely out of the picture, but my phone bill was somewhat regrettable...strangely enough, a normal salary lasts just hardly until the end of the month, let alone being sick and all day home.
But even this was something I learned to better understand, day by day. I just had to stop compensating my desperation, fear, loneliness and emptiness with shopping.

Slowly, I started regaining my self-esteem.

In November, the physiotherapist started sticking me in the "sports machine room" of his office. I began with 40 pounds on the leg press: An immense weight at the time. I was only bound to make a few repetitions; still I was completely drenched in sweat every time I exercised.

There, I met a nice lady named Andrea. It turned out she was a fellow in misery. Who else would there be in such rooms anyway?! She had problems in the cervical spine. 16 months earlier she had come on crutches because she couldn't walk on her own. "He" had freed her from the crutches. When we used to talk about our physiotherapist, we only referred to him with "He" or "Him". "He" can sometimes be rough, hits the nerve, stirs suppressed heartaches and provokes the patient in order to trigger a counter-reaction. And it worked. "He" knew exactly what "he" was talking about, what "he" may provoke, or may not.

Oh yes, I can almost see your frown, dear reader; you probably think it is obvious for a patient to become reliant on his therapist and fixed on him. Everyone who suffered such pain goes through these phases. Therapists can quickly turn to people we desperately need. It is up to the pain patient to grow beyond such feelings. But at that stage, it still was too early for me to realize that, way too early... I only know this now, five years later. I persevered stubbornly in order to buildup my muscles. I had learned and understood, that only a toned strong muscle corset can stabilize wavering vertebrae (in medical terms known as "unstable"); Oh, pardon! I meant to "keep them in their right position". All the experts told me I had to hang on in there, otherwise I would end up in a wheel chair. I understood it for good! I got it! It became my inseparable grinning companion, teased me every time I grew tired or slackened off: "Ha, I am going to get you". This idea brought me every time back to full power in the blink of an eye.

Oh no, those two wheels are not going to get me that easy. I am going to fight, as long as I can!!

My daily schedule included morning exercise at home, then going to work, returning home, taking a walk, preparing something to eat, going to the physiotherapist, relaxing, reading and conversations with the neighbors. When I went out on my usual walks, I met quite many of my neighbors, even those who lived somewhat farther away. They talked to me, they told me I could walk remarkably good now. Oh yes, to my astonishment they said they had seen and pitied me, the young woman who was so sick.

Through my walks I reached out to more and more people. November went by, and I spent my birthday with quite a few people. The weather kept getting colder; December was just around the corner, then I was sent to a cure and rehabilitation center in the "Allgäu".

Oh, I completely forgot to mention that, in September, I had to visit an examining doctor appointed by health insurance companies (or so). I was examined yet again and a meeting was conducted. Finally, based on the overall picture, the treatment at a health resort was approved. If only I knew beforehand, what a ride that was going to be…

I declined, because I didn't know if I could ever endure or even survive such a long trip (of approximately 200 miles). So the doctors decided I had to be transported lying down. But I stuck to my stand; I just couldn't do it yet, but maybe in a couple of months, and even then I wouldn't want to go to a simple "mud-baths clinic". I needed much more than that.

I tried some speed walking. It was quite difficult but proved efficient. My muscles learned to coordinate, to play in team,
to react harmonically along with my need to move forward. Every muscle was being trained, from hair to toe. In the meantime, I could also lift 80 pounds with both legs on the leg press, I could even sit in the back trainer without thinking exclusively about the pain I suffered from sitting… and managed to exercise.
The number of sports machines I used grew steadily.
A few first muscles slightly started to show… and I thought only bodybuilders could have such beautifully defined muscles. Guess what! I was wrong! Even I developed a few little pretty muscle groups. My arms and legs became stronger.
And … deep in my heart I understood I had to keep training until the end of my days, I may never neglect training, otherwise I am sure to end up in a wheel chair…
I suffered a setback of many weeks on my achieved training schedule due to a severe flu. I relentlessly thought: Never give up, hanging on in there, don't slacken off and the pain will never grow to extremes again! Just keep moving!

Dear reader, at this point you would probably say that no one should be forced to do anything. True! But what else would you do if you were in my shoes??? The wheel chair was an imminent danger, prowling right behind the corner, waiting to snatch me as soon as I stop training. Not my preferred life style…

I dreamt of a life free from pain, a life I could lead as I please, able to move freely, and I was willing to give everything for it. I discovered nevertheless, that less pain doesn't automatically mean more happiness. Only now – in May 2002 – I became able to write my story from its beginning. You are going to realize, that it still took me quite some time to write everything down. I reconciled with the pain, and first of all, with myself. That is why I wrote that saying at the end of the book. Oh no, don't sneak!

In the meantime – thanks to the pain clinic – I took part in pain-coping-strategies-training conducted by a Taiwanese psychologist. She was working on a project comparing pain patients in Taiwan and Germany. The project was back then unfortunately still in its early beginnings – and I lost contact to her. I hope to find out the project's results some day. At this point I would like to say, it is important to always be curious, to be always interested in what is going on and to take part in it… Now, back to the training: Mrs. Li explained us the mechanisms of how chronic pain originates and how we can cope with it, or better yet, master it. She taught us various relaxation methods, such as PMR (Progressive Muscle Relaxation) as developed by Jacobsen, dreaming and imaginary journeys, self-massage. One thing particularly stayed engraved in mind, namely a number of pictures assembled into a big whole, just like in a comic. The caption says:

- Enjoy yourself consciously
- Don't leave your pleasure to coincidence alone
- Take your time
- Indulge yourself with a treat
- Teach your senses on pleasure
- Better a little, but the better
- Enjoy the little things in daily life
- Enjoy yourself your way

These words are hanging in my room, I see them every day, sometimes I don't even notice them, but some other times, I read them carefully and find myself reminded of my day-to-day task: Enjoying. At the end of the course, I spoke one last time to the trainer. At the very end, she looked me in the eyes and said: "I can see it in your eyes, you will make it!" Her words still ring in my ears till this day, over and over again and they always keep me motivated.

The year 1997 drew to its end. Sometimes, I took my camera along on my speed-walking tours, I slowly started enjoying my hobby again; and that was a sign indicating I was psychologically recovering.

A car seat and its consequences

I started looking for some assistive equipment, since travelling was part of my job (doing external sales and consulting), trying to rearrange the driver's seat to suit me best. I was befallen with extreme pain every time I sat longer than half an hour in the car, which exposed the lower part of the spinal canal to pressure. How was I supposed to find a suitable seat, how much would it cost and who sells any such seats?

The health insurance company denied me its help on providing a car seat, they said I should talk to the pension insurance fund, the BfA (the German Federal Insurance Institution for Employees). Yet another association to become acquainted with. In December I filled out the necessary form, of 21 pages, to apply for an adapted car seat with several adjustment possibilities. It was quite difficult to find an appropriate distributor. But I finally found one on the southern "Weinstrasse". I soon realized that „Recaro"-made seats were nothing for me! Why did test-sitting just have to be so painful! The "ride" turned into torture.

But all hope was not lost yet, the "König" company (also known as "Formula König" mostly for car racing amateurs) had just released a completely new car seat, named something like "Rehamed" or so. It could be upholstered with individual cushions, and a hole can be made at the point where my spine is supposed to lie on the seat. It took me quite some time, but I finally gathered every cent I could get to pay the price of that seat. In the meantime, the BfA had refused my application, and to top it all off, asked me how I could "dare" buy such a seat without asking permission first. I started asking myself in which world these people actually lived.

At the same time I battled with the BfA about the kind of treatment I needed. I was bluntly told on the phone, that I am unable to evaluate my disease myself; consequently, I was allegedly unable to determine which kind of therapy may be necessary for me. Well, pain is no disease. I felt my blood boiling with anger. If only I could withdraw from this association. What am I paying since 20 years dues for, and since I don't know how long anymore, I've even been paying the maximum penalty – oh excuse me – I mean the maximum rate. Why the hell do I have to pay them dues if I don't even have the right to a minimum of reimbursement!? I am the one who had to go through hell. They are the ones standing in the way of my recovery! I have to do everything myself, why me?! A good friend of mine, suffering a hemiplegic paralysis, told me that the BfA didn't want to pay his car anymore because his doctor allegedly couldn't disclose any further information regarding him. He could have recovered. Rubbish, he just changed the doctor. After that, I heard about quite many tricks of the BfA. Aren't they human or what?

I was to be sent to a mud-bath treatment institution. This treatment clinic had only one additional special feature: cooking lessons. I already can cook, thank you. Upon serious consideration, I also knew what could be adjusted in the kitchen to suit disabled persons. But I was not "disabled" and I wasn't labeled with a disability level, no, I "just" suffer incessant pain!

We finally agreed to another postponement. On Monday, January 26, 1998 I went without a doctor's note and without rehabilitation notice…to work the normal seven hours a day.
I was so proud!
About 01:00 p.m., news circulated about our company being bought by another one. It has been seven months since the

tyrannizing pain had occupied my life. I was bewildered by the news. Eight years ago, I chose this company as employer among all others, and I wanted to keep working for it until the day I retire.

This idea about me sticking to the same employer until I retire was yet another faded hope. I went to my physiotherapist in time for my regular treatment and training. As I entered the waiting room – as usual, a couple of many many minutes too early– the physiotherapist looked at me and said "you can go straight to the treatment room"… where I let my tears flow free. Nothing was more important to him than bringing me to relax, calm down, listen to my heart and concentrate, so he skipped the regular manual therapy that day. With great difficulty I tried to accept the thought, that "we" have been bought. I had never expected this fate for our beloved company, ever. But it was the bitter truth.

At the same time, I was also negotiating with the car dealer the possibility he takes back my leased car ahead of time, though, according to the contract, I was to keep it one more year. I was undeniably stunned as the dealer said: "that's absolutely no problem; I can see what you are going through. Let us try a minivan and see whether it would be easier for you to get in and out of it and whether you find it comfortable, then we'll see about the rest". Three weeks later the new car was delivered; the dealer could make use of a contract option and managed to get the car about four weeks ahead of the usual time. Changing the leasing contract was a piece of cake. The new car was also equipped with the new car seat soon afterwards. Finally, I could drive almost painlessly to work. Well, that's quite a bit of an exaggeration, but I was just so happy about being able to take again part in normal life, about being considered a normal person again… well, I had all the necessary equipment now, but didn't get a single cent from the health insurance company or the BfA. I was guilty of making an own initiative...

My lawyer painfully tried to battle us a way through, but just couldn't achieve any progress, the car seat had costed me approximately 3000 dollars.

Yes, I know, many people would be glad not to have to go to work. Not to have to torture themselves daily with their disliked job, in an uncomfortable business stressed atmosphere. I used to feel the same way too, but having to stay seven months long home due to sickness was just too much for me. After all, I was ill; I was deprived of laughter, movement...even of the freedom to take my own decisions. I think, no illness has yet been invented, where the ill do well and are able to do whatever they want. I wanted to get back to work at all costs, to be a whole person, to prove myself ... whatever this may mean.

My chef-chef (short for: the superior of my superior) thoughtfully told me he was planning to transfer me to another position because my situation was hindering me from fulfilling the job requirements as necessary for our department. He considered it best to give me a desk-job allowing me to sit down comfortably. But for the time being, I was supposed to take the necessary cure...

I could almost cry my eyes out: the one thing that didn't suit me at all was sitting down in a chair all the time. Does this man have any idea what he is saying or doing, at all? Fortunately, letters cannot convey sound, otherwise dear reader, you would need ear-plugs. All that lack of comprehension and sensibility almost drive me to scream... Scream!!!

Treatment or rehabilitation...?

Once again I was summoned to treatment on short notice, once again I had turned down the mud-bath cure in "Allgäu", and after much quarrel, I was allowed admission into another clinic about 80 miles away from home, I could go there by car and I was supposed to begin with the treatment sometime about the end of April 1998. Because the final consent was only given at the beginning of April, I happened to be busy preparing my departure on Easter.

The day of departure finally came: Wednesday, April 29, 1998. "Please be at 01:00 p.m. on the tick here". "Of course I will". "Being punctual is what I do best". Well, soon afterwards, the chaos broke out. I was supposed to carry my luggage by myself up into my room, the same luggage I didn't even manage to carry into the car, back home. There was no parking lot free for me, although I had expressly requested to have one reserved. So I had to park my car along some roadside in the neighborhood. So I thought "Great! What a great start!" I met a nice person at the reception who transported my luggage on a trolley to my room, finally. Meanwhile I was informed that my doctor didn't have any more time for my initial examination on that day. Why am I here then? I felt myself sold down the river and couldn't stop myself from crying my eyes out the whole day long. "Lunch?" "No, it was not planned, but if you hurry up, you might find some leftovers in the kitchen". Where am I here please?

The doctor passed by in the afternoon, to bid me welcome at least. She told me, as if to comfort me, that other patients also came in today, that she wanted to examine them first, which wouldn't take much time because they just had routine tests. She said I was one of the two patients who needed more attention, which is why she will only begin with the examinations tomorrow morning. She wants to dedicate more time to the both of us. In the meantime I should unpack.

Innumerable questions popped in my mind. Routine? Care? Last in the row? When were they planning to begin with the treatment and so on, which only is possible after the initial examination. Friday happened to be May 1st, Saturdays and Sundays are off days anyway. So, what am I doing here? Unpack? Why would I do that? My boiling blood was crying out pure denial! I didn't want to sit there another minute, all I wanted was to go home!

But something happened then, as if to show that I was in the right place after all. Amidst my anger and boredom, I browsed through some event-calendars and fliers. A leaflet I just wanted to throw away caught my attention with the text imprinted on its verso: Sign Language Course. That's what I set on top of my to-do-list: getting enrolled in this course. But I didn't want to stay. What a difficult decision to make! Finally, I decided to stay. The sign language course costed much effort to take place, but it was my personal "Highlight of day" for two weeks long.

And yes, dear reader, the doctor examined me soon afterwards and actually found a few other cures I could have on that day, in addition to one or two cures for Saturday.

On the holiday of May 1st, a friend of mine living in "Cologne" came to "Wiesbaden" to pay me a visit. I was so happy to see someone dear where I felt so terribly lonely. Miserable as I was afterwards, I tried to call my pain therapist, but sadly I tried to reach him in vain. I so dearly hoped to get connected with anyone from the palliative care team, again in vain. There was no one at reach.

At some stage I broke free of my despair, I don't know how, but I did it. In the meantime, a few of us patients had started building a nice little group around the table; a group of 2 men and 4 women. The women were each respectively a year older than the other (aged 40/41/42/43), the men were nevertheless older (one was in his early 50s and the other in his mid 60s). So there we were in the spotlight because we always went out together, whether to the theater or to restaurants, to the Casino or to promenades in town... We always came up with some idea. Besides, we laughed and talked to each other a lot... and became the center of envious attention.

One of the ladies, „Uli", „my" stewardess, came across me one morning in our corridor and just took me in her arms to comfort me. It was a wonderful feeling.
The (almost) daily sport therapy built up my muscles very fast, in addition to water gymnastics, swimming, walking and stretching. There were even relaxation baths.

What was best about the treatment time? My only responsibilities were practically bathing, getting dressed and undressed, eating in the dining hall and going to bed. Let alone training, taking part at some nutrition education and some talking cures. But above all, not to forget, was the sign language course. I had all the time to take care about my own well-being, exclusively!

There was also a weird episode: once I was lying on the floor of my room, carefully training my core muscles using a heavy book. Suddenly, I heard someone knock at the door and enter immediately into the room – it was the head physician on round. Well, not quite the worse that could happen. I was praised for my diligence in exercising and the progress I had already made, somehow the conversation lead the sign language course. The Head Physician asked to see the documents related to the course, and he borrowed them. I only got them back several days later. It was the teacher who explained this behavior later on: she was served notice from the management because of a text she had made up to help us practice the sign language. That text was about a romance at a health resort, which the management didn't like at all. No, how pathetic of you, doctor… it's also a pity that I thought that doctor had a little more sense of humor, but it seems this was not a virtue he was bestowed. Laughter is the best cure, but is there any doctor who ever learns this?

We laughed much in the sign language course, because we somehow were clumsy at using our hands, although they are our daily work-tool. There we were missing the nuances, negligent of the right moves, and our teacher "Conny" explained that we just conveyed a message completely different than the one intended. We learned MCL (Manually Coded Language) instead of DGS (German Sign Language). The difference between them: the MCL is a sign translation of each word as spoken in common language, the DGS on the other hand, has its own grammar and syntax, it is a language of its own.
The days went by… my partner wanted to pay me a visit one day, his room was booked but he fell ill and couldn't come to visit. Instead my parents came to see me, they too had to endure a long ride to see me. But then we got comfortable in town. Thanks to my car, equipped with a special seat, I was quite easily on the move, independent and could drive much about, which otherwise would not have been possible. What else should I do, when the last treatment session ends at 02:00 p.m.?

I even found chances to shoot a few photographs.

The month of May brought along a quite hot weather, the temperature rose to over 86°F. Obviously, the clothes I had packed for three weeks were all somewhat too warm. Right! There were malls in Wiesbaden… and they ought to earn some money from my expenditures.

All in all, I was happy about the way those three weeks went by. Two of them were really filled with treatments, most of which I could also had done in the comfort of my home, but not this intensively. Sometimes I feel the need to take some time for myself again, to only take care of me and of my body and let everything else take its natural flow. So be it, life carried a completely different surprise for me, but more about that at the end of the story. All that matters is that I found a friend there, "Uli"–"my stewardess". We battled courageously through life supporting each other as much as we only could. This reminds me of a summer-hot weekend.
She was bare foot, but was so excited to greet my parents that she rushed to meet them on the sidewalk and had to jump from one foot to the other because the floor was so hot she couldn't stand.

When I look back at that time, I can say that the treatment provided me at least with more confidence about the way to treat my body. I know my limits now, and my potentials. Unfortunately, I stopped exercising backstroke swimming and forgot the method by now, I am not quite a water dog anyway.

I enjoy contemplating the water, whether the waves of a beach, of a sea or of a rivulet in the woods…it always fills me with peace… I sincerely enjoy the moments I spend along the water.

One last glance back at pain management:
During the course I kept thinking "what's that supposed to lead to, I already know all these things". Now I know there is a great difference between knowing and understanding on one hand, and taking that knowledge to heart on the other... just like almost everything in life. Yes, seriously now! Even philosophizing is part of pain management! It helps us find our place again in this world, accept that place and embrace it.

A year later

I was particularly happy with growing able to get by without painkillers, every once in a while I just needed something against headaches, just like everybody else. I finally managed to keep my pain under control thanks to physical and muscle training.
That's correct, your eyes didn't play any tricks on you; you really just read "keep under control". At the time, I was still far from being able to come to terms with the pain; the pain and I had rather come to a peaceful coexistence whereby each of us would grant the other enough space to live on. No, no, it takes time to master such a situation, the fitting saying goes: "Patience! With time grass becomes milk."

Or like this poem:

On Pain
By Katrin A. Kling

Dreams were made to be
Made to flow through me
Destined to resist pain
Nearly setting me from life in twain
The miraculous cure has a name Lidocain.

Pain, nagging at my soul mercilessly
Pain, my companion constantly
Pain, what is it you want with me?
How long must I endure thee?
Pain, I despise you
Why, why come to me?

Pain, my endless nightmare
Do I have no other choice
than your presence to bear?

Won't you ever fade away?
If you are meant to persist
I am doomed to go astray.

Pain, my archenemy
I've so often shed tears
So dearly wishing you'd set me free
But you insist sticking on to me
Pain, won't you ever go away?
Are you trying to become a friend?
Or am I first to face my end?

Should I see you as a friend?
Should we even form a band?
Do you happen to know a song?
Maybe I could sing along.
Pain, you are more than I can take.

Summer began and we decided to go on vacation. But where? I was not yet able to endure a long drive. We actually wanted to go to Switzerland again. Then, we remembered we once went to Lake Biel four years ago and stayed at a wonderful hotel. So we called the hotel and it turned out that the room we had back then was available; so we booked the room for six days only, just out of precaution.

We spent a great vacation. We enjoyed our time and visited wonderful places; even the Butterfly Garden of Tignes was opened, renovated and larger. It had burnt down some time earlier. Now, there was even a nocturnal animals' garden harboring living and freely flying animals. Fascinating!

As we came back on August 22nd, I knew I had to take the next step on the path of my professional education. My new field of expertise was entitled: "SAP EarlyWatch". The training lasted 10 weeks, of which I skipped the first because my familiarity with SAP was already four years of age. This was no piece of cake; most of the participants were remarkably younger than me. But I balanced this out with my professional expertise. In the meantime, there were clients insisting on seeing me. Unfortunately, they lived very far from the main railway line, which made it relatively harder to reach them. But I finally did; after all, it was a violation of my codex to let the client have me picked at home up at his own expense – by a cab.

By the end of October, the training phase had also passed by. So I returned to normal deskwork. It was fairly okay. Frictions with my superiors crept into day-to-day life, my contact to customers gradually became regular again and the relocation chaos began. We relocated four times within seven months. The quantity of my belongings in the office shrunk from about 40 cartons to six by our arrival to the last location, now I only had two cartons of work-material left. The more I cleared out on the outside, the more I felt free. A great deal of developments took place in the time between November 1998 and October 1999. Meanwhile, I oversaw that my love life was falling to pieces and that I only had a few carefully selected friends left; friends who lived as far away from me as possible.

You might be amazed by the realizations I made... Oh, yes, my perception ability can be quite astounding, especially when it comes to three- or four-year-old happenings. At that time distance, everything was "no problemo".

More and more tasks were referred to me on the job, starting with the application of what I had learned. Once, for example, during a sales consultation, I was required to take the customer's database into consideration based on the given rules of salesmanship and deduct from it all essential arguments for the conversation with the customer, in addition to conducting a qualified consulting session. Much high praise and a flourishing business were the result, though not always as originally planned, but still lucrative for my employer. I intensified my work with our hardware suppliers, the partnership with whom I had helped establish in the late 1996.

Part II – Words of Contemplation

You want to be loved,
because you do not love,
but the moment
you love,
it is finished,
you are no longer inquiring
whether or not
somebody loves you.

Krishnamurti

Words from the Depths of my Exhaustion

One particular phase of my life carried along many setbacks; it was so bad that I temporarily needed tranquilizers that also had a positive effect on my severe pain. Pain came by, every now and again, claiming time and space. I studied it over the years, observed it with much self-awareness.
Then I understood: it is important...essential...vital for me to know my limits and abide by them, to challenge myself without overstraining it.
And: to set a limit to myself and to others and take care, that they comply with them, that they respect and accept me, as a I am.

I am still learning, it is an endless process. As long as we humans live, we have something to learn. This kind of learning must be coupled with courage, much courage. This truth is even anchored in common belief: whoever takes the path of learning never comes to its end, never grows up, never has anything to say. It must have once been essential to come to an end with learning at a certain point, because it meant "finding one's place in life". These values have only a minor importance in modern fast moving society. What really matters nowadays is to understand ourselves, to understand where we truly belong to. Then, we will automatically find our rightful place, whether in society or anywhere around the world.

Therefore, it is necessary to keep our eyes open, to remain vigilant, to restructure our way of thinking; it is necessary to be ready to change our points of view. There was much talk, in the last few years, about the so-called "Paradigm shift". This here is not much different: changing a point of view and shifting a paradigm.

Some time ago, I saw a poster hanging in the social service institution, picturing a blue elephant lying down on his back and raising his trunk aloft. At a closer look I realized a mole was sitting on the edge of the trunk and "changing perspective". Follow the example of this little mole: Have the courage to discover new sights, new readings, new thoughts.

Rüdiger Dahlke and Louise L. Hays showed us new thinking and perspectives in their writings years ago. No one owns the absolute truth, but they taught us to see the world through new eyes. No matter which religion or dogma you adhere to, don't shy away from taking off the glasses you are seeing the world through. Look at yourself, at your world and your pain through new eyes. If you need more suggestions, you can find them in the works of Dahlke, Hays or of Wolf-Dieter Storl, or you could opt for exploring different cultures such as the Chinese or Indian culture. When it comes to cultures, please keep in mind that each of them is unique and original. Many treatment methods and therapies are only helpful because they are rooted in culture and beliefs. It would be no use to apply them isolated from their original mystical environment.

Learn to understand yourself and your body; but above all, learn to accept yourself, your body and even your pain. Put an end to your struggle against the pain and against yourself.

Accepting means letting go. Only when you accept your pain, you become able to let it go.

Then, you probably won't need the pain anymore to

- draw attention to yourself,
- be noticed,
- get around something you do not want to do
- accept yourself as you really are

Here, an example of a world without pain. Some time ago, I met a lady having trouble with her new glasses. The doctor told her to wear glasses and contact lenses alternately. Her cornea was strongly damaged and the doctor urged her to increasingly rely on glasses. She told me she repudiated wearing glasses her whole life long; she didn't want to admit her "weakness", and always wore contact lenses instead. As we brought up, at some point of the conversation, that she now must concede this weakness or otherwise loose her eyesight, she became thoughtful. Her struggle with her weakness brought her continuously in trouble.
In conclusion: only when she accepts herself with all the bad and the good, she will live in peace, even with her eyes.

Words breaking free from me

I kept my story caged in my heart for a very long time, the truth be said, I carried it around ever since 1997. It lasted even longer until I started writing down bits of it. Typing took only two nights' time; it was late May 2002. Afterwards, I took a break, and then I started writing a few nights over again.

During the summer of 2003, I began a new life and a new career as independent consultant (Adlerian holistic psychology) and trainer of people new to computers. I am still self employed till this day, as Adlerian holistic psychological consultant, as executives' coach in small and medium-sized enterprises, as communication trainer and speaker. Since I am creative and always on the move, I also take part in projects beyond this frame, like writing a book for instance, or articles for newspapers or on the internet.

Seven years long, I coached a local self-help group on Pain, but I stopped in the meantime, and I give speeches every now and then about pain and its management, but also about other subjects such as letting go, setting limits and self-acceptance. The nucleus of my consulting changed.

Many other things in my life changed as well. In 2012, I let go of everything, each and every thing that needed to be let go of. By the end of the year, I reached a point in my life where nothing was still as it once was. An entirely new life is ahead. It is slightly

frightening, but nothing can shade off my curiosity and entrepreneurial spirit.

Life goes on. And I learn something new every day. Erik Blumenthal once said: "there is no one from whom I cannot learn anything, and there is no one who cannot learn anything from me." In this sense, have a happy learning!

Conciliating words: Pain therapist and Pain patient

Coaching chronic pain patients can be marked with many misunderstandings, wrong expectations and time shortage at the crowded doctor's office. This is why both doctor and patient are frustrated most of the times.

Not very long ago, a 83-years-old pain patient came in while I was speaking from stage. He sat in the first row and asked his questions like everybody else. He said he's been suffering since the end of World War II due to an accident resulting in a broken thoracic vertebra. The doctors didn't listen to him, they just sent him away because he was allegedly only "imagining" the pain. After my speech he approached to talk to me. Before he left, he said: "Thank you very much for the speech, and most of all for listening to me." Can you imagine the shock of hearing such words from the lips of an 83-year-old man?!

He experienced everything pain patients usually suffer on their odyssey through doctors' offices. He went through his decades-long odyssey, visited innumerable doctors, put up with being called a pretender… and didn't find anyone who really listened to him. This must be the reason why he was not provided with any suitable medical care.

The list of feelings and shortcomings of a pain patient is long:

- They feel alone and lonely.
- They do not feel associated.
- They feel patronized and infantilized, because they are deprived of everything (mainly by the closest family

members), in other words, no one takes them seriously even when everything is on its usual course
- They completely lose confidence in themselves, because everyone else loses confidence in them.
- They lose the ability to make decisions and plans, because others start making decisions for them.
- They are aimless, all that counts is the next moment without pain; so they stop planning their future.
- They feel misunderstood because no one listens to them.
- They feel angry, because their lives are being lead by others and because the endless good-meant paternalism is depriving them of the slightest chance to live their own lives.
- Not their illness is the problem, but their life.

Burdened with such feelings, the majority of pain patients visit the doctor filled with way too high expectations, namely wishing for nothing but complete freedom from pain. But this is feasible only in the rarest cases, soothing the pain on the other hand is more realistic and can be achieved.

But the expectations don't end here; the patients expect the doctor to act like a magician, HE has to do it, HE has to wipe the pain away. At first, the patients don't show any personal initiative. They mostly face the doctor displaying their body language. Upon talking to the patient about taking an initiative, I mostly get slammed with an answer like: "Yes, I've already visited so many doctors". No, no, this is not what I meant with "initiative". But, more about this later.

How can the relation, the attitude between therapist and patient be changed? What can each do?

The empathy of both therapist and patient should come to light. Both parties must open up to each other, they must understand that they have come together in order to ease the pain with their joined forces and knowledge. This is, on the one hand, based on the therapist's capacity to listen to his patient very carefully, in addition to him being honest, open and encouraging. The patient has the right to be taken seriously and to enjoy the complete of attention of his therapist. The key to the decisive difference of giving the patient the feeling of being heard, lies in granting him just a few minutes longer; instead of 3, 5 minutes he could be given 4!

There are no standard patients. Pain patients are so multifaceted and diverse as life itself.

The patient must be encouraged and motivated to make own initiatives, in order to begin with the first step of a long journey; in other words, he needs to be encouraged to gather information regarding his own medical case, to look for new movement possibilities, to relax and start to act.
Communication on an equal basis between the patient and his doctor is essential. When the doctor stops being intimidated by well-informed patients, when he even encourages them to gather information, then, half the work is practically done.
The patient, on the one hand, needs to keep his decision-making ability, and to be supported in this matter.
Discouragement is taboo for both parties. The doctor refrains from using words such as "simulating", "pretender" or "you are beyond therapy, no one can help you" and the patient stays friendly and sticks to his questions.
Another necessity is patience and endurance of both, as well as staying strong.

I am well aware of the fact that well-informed patients are still an intimidation to doctors; although they, of all people, have the best chances to heal. All they need is a little support and a helping hand so that they may take, and remain, on the right path. So, dear patients and dear doctors, stay strong! Each person has the right to strike out a new path and learn something new. And when two people do this together, it's all the better.

And when you, as patient, come to the point of saying: "I can handle my pain, not the other way round" you know that a new life is beginning and that it is up to you to mold it.

Part III – From pain patient to pain person. Become your own coach.

A word on implementation

It's a long journey. The road is steep, stony and complicated. This may sound quite discouraging. We feel ourselves alone most of the time, exhaust ourselves with vain battles and fail to find new strengths. We get lost within our selves, forgetting that out there, there are people who would really like to help. They just don't know how. We need to guide them, to tell them how in order to grow in life, to let them in to our world controlled by pain. Most patients experience others as a "dominant", feel themselves damned to faineance, get filled with sadness, with anger, and feel deeply misunderstood.

Through my own story with pain, you have seen a demonstration of how the typical life of a pain patient develops, you saw the beginning of pain, into the pain, the chronification, the withdrawal from normal life, the fear from the future, fear to do anything, fear of planning anything, fear to move, fear of going out among people, fear of rejection, fear of loneliness... This ever-present fear ravages self-confidence, confidence in one's own strengths, the courage to turn to others and even the need to take part in life.
This is how cocooning starts, which originally is a vogue catch-word referring to persons who draw back from social into domestic life avoiding human contact and ceasing participation in social life.

But there always is a chance to move again, to re-take part in social life, to feel part of something and put an end to loneliness. My story depicted nothing else; it was all about Pain – Withdrawal – Return.

Each stage has its own characteristics and each of them requires special capacities. The most important part however, is to take a look back and see the possibilities. Let me put it in other words: "Falling down" is nothing to be ashamed of, but "staying down" is. So, always stand up again when you fall. Don't let the circumstances mislead you, forge your own circumstances instead, mold your own life. You are the only one who knows what you really need, what makes you feel better. Make your decisions yourself and don't let yourself be influenced by anyone else. You can, of course, seek advice from specialists, more experienced peers or even good friends. But taking the decision on what is beneficial for you, what may help you or have a positive influence on your life, is something only you should, can and must do.

At this point, I would like to wish you many good advisors, just as many advisors and jesters as had the Kings of the east and west. They listened to their advisors, but made their decisions alone, based on their acquired knowledge and their own intelligence, and they stood up for their decisions.

Hereunder, you will find a description of a method to set yourself free from pain. Each person is unique and goes her own way, whether old or young, man or woman… Consider everything in the description below as an offer. Try to follow my lead; after all, actions speak louder than words! And you just happen to be holding a book of the series having the same title, namely: "Actions speak louder than words". There is much you can read and learn about this subject, but the most of it will probably remain latent in your memory, waiting to come into application, which never happens. Based on my own experience, I allow myself to constantly remind you of the necessity to become active and to put into practice what you read. So: "Actions speak louder than words…I mean your own actions, practicing what you learned, experienced, read and heard."

P.S: I am writing this chapter lying in a canvas chair of my terrace in the sunshine. I learned to find what best suits me in the light of the circumstances. By the way, the neighbor's cat seems to be very attached to me: she either lies near to me between the flowers of my backyard or under my car, practicing "active relaxation". At the moment it is quite loud and busy inside her home because of the many cheerful ladies who came to visit. Whenever I forget to look after my needs, I just take a look at that cat. She shows me, time and time again, how important it is to take care of one's self. Two more years have already passed, and I am still taking care of myself, like for instance by going spontaneously on vacation at Lake Garda. The restaurant I sat in, known as "Al Gabbiano" (The Seagull) on recommendation of a good friend who's a regular guest here when on business trips to "Marmor" in Veneto. He was absolutely right, only one restaurant could keep up with its level of quality and that's the „Caffè degli Artisti" in the "Verona Arena". Surely it doesn't have the same stylish surrounding views with white tablecloths and elegant service, but it is very peaceful, has an original Italian atmosphere and an excellent cuisine. I just love it. Part of my recovery process was to find out what suits me best, such as the things I mentioned above.

One more thing occurs to me here: appreciation, honor and mutual respect are becoming ever rarer in this modern hurried lifestyle and performance stress. Chronically ill patients are thus part of the most disadvantaged, always faced with something like: "Don't be silly, come on, you can make it, it can't be all that bad…"

It is always good to gather information and stay up-to-date, but as long as that knowledge remains only in your mind, it is just a useless encumbrance. Only practicing it leads to benefits. It reveals how much you've understood of what you read. What you read or learned was maybe not suitable for your case, but rather just a series of embellished words. The words you read were maybe not the right ones for you… or so. Finally, the decisive measure is the one that usually lacks, namely taking action.

It is thus very, very, very important that you take action, otherwise all those words will remain hollow, blown away by the merest breeze and sentenced to be forgotten. At the moment, I can only ascertain the following:

- You want to change something for your own sake.
- You are the most important person in your life.
- You deserve the improvement of your quality of life.

Grasp your rightful portion, grant yourself an improvement, take action. You know what is best for you!

So, get going.

Starting at this point, I will be introducing the program dedicated to pain patients. Search herein for whatever suits and comforts you. Always keep in mind that you absolutely must carry on and persevere, not only in your mind, but in daily life as well. This is the only way for you to achieve a beneficial change and a new beginning with the management of your pain.
I shall use the LISA-method to point up a few things.

It's my playground

You must have been asking yourself all the time: when does she come to the point, when does the program start? How am I finally going to get started?

It sounds so easy…although it is the most difficult part of all. You begin with yourself, with your pain… I know it doesn't sound much inviting, but there is no way you can avoid this step. A friend of mine reacted a few weeks ago with panic to this statement, saying: "No, no, no, I don't want to know anything about me, my body or my illness. It scares me…"

Begin with asking yourself the following question: "How am I doing today, how am I doing right now?" Listen to your inner self, into the deepest depths of your soul, until you feel there is nothing more to be heard, there is only darkness and the end of the world. What do you hear? What are your body, your soul and your mind discussing right now? Oh, you don't understand the language they're speaking? Well, not yet. Sit back, relax and listen carefully. Just listen. Don't do anything else in the meantime, don't let yourself be distracted with anything else, stay relaxed and calm and listen "what's up" inside of you. Doing this more often whilst retiring from the world's noises, will allow you someday to hear your inner dialogue. Let yourself be surprised by the emerging secrets.

Relaxation

Do you have difficulties concentrating on yourself alone?
In this case, it is high time to resort to relaxation methods. Do you know any? Have you ever tried any? Then it is long overdue. I relax when I contemplate the waters for hours and hours, whether from ship or shore, clearing my mind of any thoughts, just letting everything flow on, not undertaking any wild actions like I usually do… just being.

You surely object now and say that relaxation doesn't work for you. Honestly now, I think you just didn't search long enough yet. Are you a rather active person? If you are, you are then going to need relaxation methods such as Progressive Muscle Relaxation or Meditative Dancing, anyhow something enclosing slow movement. You can't bear autogenic training or silent meditation. Such methods were rather conceived for passive people who don't really like movement. What best suits them are still and quiet meditative relaxation methods.

Are you surprised? This question actually was subject of a pain research study because relaxation methods failed to help many pain patients. Later, it was found out that there are active and passive people – or at least roughly grouped. And each of these two groups responds to different methods. I hope you are feeling somewhat better understood now.

By the way: I am basically an active person, still, I sometimes enjoy autogenic training or simple self-awareness exercises, both are rather passive methods. So, don't let yourself be squeezed into a pattern. Instead, examine carefully which type of person you are and begin with the corresponding relaxation exercises. After you start mastering them, continue to look for other ways and measures that make you feel good. Don't be afraid to try something new.

A last brief notice about active and passive people: active people are those who get informed and move straight away to the application, they don't hesitate long before getting to action. They are the fidgeters, the restless, the decision-makers and action-takers. They take action in spite of any consequences, even if it turns out, they were entirely wrong, they still take action.

Passive people on the other hand, are rather hesitating; they hem and haw 3-5 times before doing or not doing something. They are rather skeptical and in extreme cases, the ones who let life pass them by, just lying around on a sofa. They let actions and decisions be taken by others for them.

This is why relaxation methods are so different. Passive people prefer autogenic training or fantasizing in contrast to active people who need movement, who need their activity even while relaxing, and thus something such as Progressive Muscle Relaxation. Still, it is interesting to know, that fantasizing seems to be suitable for both kinds of people.

Now, you need to find out whether you are a passive or an active person, or perhaps a bit of both. To the latter: Congratulations, you are the biggest winner of all, you can benefit from all kinds of techniques, so dive into the great knowledge of relaxation methods.

At this point, I would like to wish you much fun and progress.

Back to me – Beginning and End

The big moment has finally come: You can hear whatever is being spoken, whispered, shouted or mumbled; you recognize the sources of angry cries and of tears. Are you surprised? Or are you somehow already familiar with such matters? With voices saying:

"Come on, relax."
"Now just take care of yourself."
"Set finally some limits and stop letting yourself be exploited."
"Stand up to yourself, don't let the others break your spirits."

Don't be frightened at such emerging expressions. The beginning lies right here. Are you afraid of where this might be leading you? Don't worry; it is only leading you back to yourself, not anywhere else. Did you notice that you are important? Only you and no one else?! You are important, you matter, you need a change, you need new ideas about the way to manage your pain. You, only you know what is going on inside of you and how to make use of your knowledge… how to apply it.

And now we come to one of the big and essential questions:

Is it okay to be selfish?

YES, it is more than just okay, it even is good. Be selfish. At this point, this is an essential realization. Be selfish. Yes, I am familiar with all objecting arguments, and I can refute them all. There is no use even trying to argue with me. In this point you can only lose, believe me. Should you have the spirit to argue anyway, please don't hesitate to contact me. My office will connect you to me straight away.

Most people think on selfishness: "ugh, bah, that's bad! I have to think of the others." Yes, of course you may think of the others, as long as you keep in mind to think of yourself AND take action for your own sake. Allow me to remark here, that this has NOTHING to do with egoism. You are probably thinking now about egomania, which is the characteristic of people who can think solely and exclusively of themselves. Such people never face the dilemma of thinking of anyone else; all they care about is themselves and their own interests and well-being…

Again: egoism is a healthy state of mind. Every human being needs this characteristic; without it he wouldn't survive. Most women were brought up to always care for others first and only last for themselves. Priority goes to the husband, children, parents, neighbors, friends, home, garden, colleagues, pets, job etc. If, in the course of a given year, 8 seconds happen to be left over for themselves, they don't know what to do of them.

Women were brought up to serve and nurture. They always care for others. Men, however, were brought up to "conquer" the world. True, this sounds too simple, and surely not highly philosophical. But, what does a look back onto your own life reveal? Aren't women rather caring and nurturing?

If you even slightly agree with me here, I would like to invite you to consider yet another approach: Women haven't really learned to take care of themselves. This is where the difficult part begins. A women's first duty, whether with or without pain, is to look after herself, tend to herself and establish her own well-being. After she pursues, fulfills and secures this goal, she can tend to everyone else without harming herself. And we can only take good care of others if we take good care of ourselves.

Well, here we come back again to those 8 seconds. Have you forgotten what you last read? In this case, please take a glance back on the last page… Learn to make good use of those 8 seconds, for a start.

One more a bit of elucidation combined with my own experience: constantly neglecting your soul and giving priority to others (whether people or things), will make your soul wilt, become miserable and finally aim to reach out to you, you just won't listen. Some day it will cry out loud, but you'll shut your inner ears to it, you don't want to hear it.
Soon comes the point where we shut our soul's mouth, we gag it to force it to silence, to force it to stop annoying or distracting us from our desire to neglect ourselves and tend to others instead. Now, we completely deny ourselves and our needs. Our body starts to suffer and sends us signals, but we deliberately look the other way. There's no time for aches and ailments. Our will controls everything.

An example

A woman, wife and mother stands by her family. She sacrifices her job, takes care of the house, the kids, the garden, maintains relations, organizes and arranges this and that and simply does everything for the family. She feels satisfied and happy at the beginning, everybody is doing well. But the kids eventually grow more and more independent, her husband seems to have built himself up another life and she doesn't feel needed anymore. She attempts a desperate try to make herself a little indispensable, but neither kids nor husband are pleased and move to the defense. Tending to house and garden gives her no sense of fulfillment. She feels lonely, disregarded and can't even express herself.

She doesn't realize yet what is going on with her – or what isn't. She starts falling ill, is plagued with little aches at first, once this, once that; anyway, she can't tend to the family. And when she can, then only does it very painfully, giving her family the feeling of guilt without knowing why. She then starts suddenly having pain. She goes through every medical instance and is checked up by different doctors, but no one can come to a clear result.

And then a diagnosis finally brings about some clarity, or so it seems. It followed by vain treatments and rehabilitation sojourns where she finally finds the time to take care of herself. Long discussions with other patients, with therapists and with her inner self bring a first awareness.

But merely three or four weeks after rehab and everything is history. The discussed measures on tending to herself are already forgotten. Everything is now going back to its old routine.

Remark

Are you alarmed by the fact that everything slipped into forgetting? This is even normal after almost each rehabilitation process, after each so furiously started training. Almost nothing is kept in mind. Even increasing training would lead to the same result. Or so it seems. This reminds of an old saying: Little strokes fell big oaks. It perfectly applies when you keep on learning. And yet we must consider that this might work only in some cases and lead to a change, mostly a positive change, but in many other cases, it takes much more time until even a slightest change comes into being, and in some others, it doesn't help at all. Unfortunately, there is a very high number of chronic pain patients who don't come to any improvement at all.

Would you like to know why? Well, think about it a little bit. Ponder again on the story I told you here above. The woman in my story needs –even if subconsciously– her pain in order to draw the others' attention to herself. If she lets go of the pain, she won't be dedicated so much attention anymore. What a fatal vicious circle!

Only then, when she chooses herself and consequently becomes able to let go of her pain, then, yes only then, she won't need the attention anymore… and the vicious circle will be broken. You can find more information in this regard in Part IV of this book under "Case Studies", which will help you to better understand.

Here we come back to: "Actions speak louder than words". Apply what you learned, keep persevering, and undertake everything that helps you break your vicious circle of pain.

The 8 golden seconds

Here we are again, I suddenly have 8 seconds all at once just for me. Well, I admit I have overplayed it a little bit. Would you have kept reading if I told you, you had eight hours for yourself? Of course not: Eight hours are a long time after all, aren't they?

Let us take a look at how this spare time can be used for just a little egoism.

I already introduced the relaxation methods. Have you already found something to suit you? No? Then it is high time to do! And no, it is never too late, it only is high time. Relaxing will help you focus a bit more on yourself and discover what is beneficial for you. This is where it gets exciting.

Since none of the following is just mental exercise, the first exercise begins now:

What do you NEED to feel good?

Take a blank piece of paper. Use only two thirds of its left part, one third of the right part will have a very particular use, so please don't use now. On the left part, write everything down that makes you feel good, one thing below the other, in form of a list. So what do you need in order to feel well?

I have a few suggestions for you: a blue sky, sunshine, bubble baths in candle light, an own garden, going out walking or jogging, a glass of wine, a tasty meal, sex, pleasant conversations, books, activities of any kind etc. Write everything down and keep your list up-to-date.

Here comes the right third of the paper into play. Consider your list as column 1, draw three additional columns next to it. The additional columns don't need to be wide, just enough to tick them off. These three columns have the following meanings:

1. Indispensable and not negotiable.
2. Important but not impossible to be conceded.
3. "nice to have" but not having it won't break my heart

I am going now to give an example on additional column no. 2: imagine you have a balcony and you want to buy yourself an awning as sunblind. It must be electrically operated, the measurement must fit, it has to be white and imprinted with red roses. You go shopping and it turns out that measurements, electric operation and the white color are all okay, all except the red-rose imprints. It only is offered with sunflower imprints. Now imagine that the indispensable characteristics were met. The color could be important, but it is not the end of the world, if you bought it with sunflower imprints. So, this means that point 2 is important to me, but I can still concede it.

And now, I bid you much fun, creativity and self-awareness in writing down your personal list and ticking off the most important choices for you.

Just a short remark about the assessment: please take a look at what you ticked off in the first column. How many of these things do you already have? How many are you lacking? Take care and indulge yourself, even if only few items of your list are at hand. Only you can do the things that make you feel good; no one else can. Alright, a massage is carried out by a masseur, but you are the one who decides you need a massage at the first place, you ask for an appointment and you go to the spa. And you even decide if the masseur has offered you a good massage or not.

What you could learn from this chapter? Learn to take good care of yourself, so that you never get confused and never let spare time for yourself just pass you by, even if that time was no longer than 8 seconds. Take provisory measures, learn for your own sake, try new things carefully and find out what makes you feel well… and when you do, always keep it in mind, always within reach.

Gathering and assessing information

Gather information and acquire all possible knowledge concerning the pain. Go to a library, ask your doctor, search the internet or refer to a self-help group.
Gather all the information to learn everything you can possibly learn about your illness. This will help you, it will make you feel better. You stop being helpless, when you know all about the illness.

I would like to guide you a little further by using an example on back pain, which in this case is in the lower back, accompanied by severe pain depriving you from sleep, hindering the slightest movement even depriving you from sit down. The learning process might be as follows:
On a random internet research, you look for the most exhaustive and fastest information resource. You come across blogs, websites of organizations such as pain organizations, of medical associations or self-help organizations. You find questionnaires about all kinds of pain, as well as tips on pain-relief on the websites of specialists etc.
You keep on groping for answers, you enter more and more keywords, describe the pain more and more precisely in your queries and all at once you enter a new world of comprehensive information. You find pictures, diagrams, texts, personal experience reports, medical reports, statistics and treatment options.

You gradually manage to narrow your symptoms' pattern down, you find out, for instance, that it was not the slipped disc that triggered the pain and the real triggers were tendons, ligaments and bad joints in the lower back which became twisted like the Sacroiliac Joint (SI) for example.

P.S: You are going to realize, what a comprehensive resource Wikipedia is, that new information is continuously added up and that its articles are up-to-date, carefully reviewed and easy to understand. When you come across technical terms you can't understand, all you have to do is click the link to open the explanation. This is how it is guaranteed that everyone can understand the published information.

Well, this is how you get further. You keep on growing wiser, you are well-informed on your pain and its circumstances. You are adapting.

I hope and wish, that you soon become as curious about yourself and your body as I was about mine. You are going to realize, what a competent conversation partner for your therapists you are going to become. You get active, take part in the conversation, because it is about you after all. Please, don't be scared by the wrong idea, that your knowledge of the functions and abilities of your own body may harm you. No, quite on the contrary: the more you know, the better you will be able to manage your situation and the better you can discern which therapy is the good and right one for you.

How are you doing? Do you feel a little better now? I am not asking just for fun. Actually, I know your pain has meanwhile pushed you into a desperate situation, that is to say the least of it.

- You are suffering,
- You are distancing yourself from your social environment
- You don't dare to make any plans anymore
- You don't feel capable of setting an appointment at farther than 24 hours
- You are retiring more and more into yourself
- You feel that the big black hole you fell into keeps growing darker
- ALL that is left of you is pain.

Did you answer to the majority of the above statements with "yes"? Look again at the list, read it one more time. How does it feel? Do you want to stay where you actually are?
Or do you want to take part again in social life?

WHAT.DO.YOU.REALLY.WANT???

Information – and what now?

You have collected so much information that your head feels about to explode, your eyes are tired from reading and you can't seem to absorb a single word of information anymore. And this is good, because it means you have already absorbed very much. Now you know almost everything about your situation and that, in words you can understand!

So what are going to do with all this knowledge?

Begin with letting it all ease off. Let it sink in. This knowledge must be allowed to find itself the right place in your mind and fill it in. The time for it to sink in is different from one person to the other. Now it is important not to rush anything. You have the right to take your time. Find your own tempo and stick to it.

P.S: Pain patients are labeled most of the time. One label is their categorization into active or passive people, as I already mentioned in the chapter on relaxation here above.
Passive patients, on the one hand, remain so long obstinate in their situation and often, too often, can't find their way out; they fail to make a change. Applied to their pain, it means, they obstinate in the pain-situation and fail to set themselves free from it, they are unevenly likely to remain pain patients throughout their entire lives.
Active people, on the other hand, don't put up long with the same situation. These are most probably the readers waiting impatiently to reach the next part of the text, longing to know what the next stage looks like. Active people look for solutions and ideas to overcome painful situations. They are curious, creative, they move

into gear and don't put up with an unpleasant situation because it stirs in them the need to change, to establish their well-being.

You surely understand now my appeal in the last pages:
Find your tempo and stick to it. Doing what? Changing, recovering

- Your quality of life
- Your courage to face life
- Your plans for the future
- Your mobility
- Your activity
- Your happiness
- Your social life, i.e.
    - Seeing friends
    - Going out to theater, movies or concerts
    - Building up relations to others
    - Living your sexuality
    - Enjoying the little things in daily life
    - Going shopping all by yourself
    - Exercising your profession

You are invited to extend, change or curtail the list as you please.

And here comes the most important question: How do you get there? How do you achieve all that?

First of all, you must figure out what each point of the above list means to you. Let us start with quality of life and mobility.

What does „quality of life" mean to you? Pursuing normal life again, being free or almost free of pain, not being restricted in your movements, taking part in social life? What does it mean to you? You surely nodded in assent to most of these statements. Did you notice how familiar I am with this situation? I know what I am talking about.

At this point, I would like to tell you what I felt like, even if I already described it in detail in the first part of this book. Back then, I ended up deprived of everything: my quality of life, my courage to face life, my mobility, my laughter, my future, my job, my sexuality, my independence and my self-determination. I felt completely useless. But as I already said, I was very lucky to have met the right therapists for me at an early stage. You must have noticed my exuberant will to live and need for movement. Both were backed up by my doctor and therapist, each through his possibilities and choices: by the doctor who talked to me and guided me to self-reflection and by the physiotherapist through adapted and systematically structured movements.

Allow me to remind you of my „conquest" of my immediate surroundings as I started walking again, first around the house, then around the block, then out in the street, until I managed to walk an entire mile – in a good 40 minutes, followed by the next victory, namely walking that one mile within only 20 minutes. The whole process took me 3 or 4 months time. The next step surely followed, I mean walking even more miles at a moderate pace. And it worked. It felt like breaking out of my chains, my muscles grew stronger, my need for movement was satisfied on the one hand, and on the other, movement was to me just like an addiction (which I only say now that 15 years have passed by).

This is what quality of life meant for me. I could move, became more resilient, was able to accomplish day-to-day tasks on my own again, at some stage I could tend to the garden, go back to work, reintegrate into society and take part in normal life. And so it was, that each step interacted with other to attract yet another pleasant progress. That was quality of life changing. I grew more responsible and didn't put up with anything so easily anymore; quite on the contrary, I sought to my well-being, but not all the time, I must admit. And I even forgot much of the knowledge I had acquired so painfully.

So, what conclusion did you draw?

What do you consider important? What is quality of life from your point of view? When you figure out the answer to this question, don't stop until you reach exactly this goal. Then, you will also be soothing your pain.

Some more ideas ...

Pain, Friends and Loneliness

You are tired of pain being the center of attention. You can't take it anymore? You would just like to cut your pain out like a piece of dead meat? All this pain is becoming for you too much to bear. This pain hindering you from taking part in life, from going to the theater or the restaurant, or even to go on vacation? Does everyone you meet ask how the pain is doing? Do you still have any friends at all? Or did most of them turn their back on you while you were barricading yourself at home only communicating through the phone? Didn't your friends want to hear anything anymore about your pain by the third time you called? Did most of them already run off?

In this case, you are facing a crossroad, whether you like or not.

You can decide whether you want your friends back or find new ones. Are you outraged? Why? Aren't both logic possibilities for you to consider? Are you angry with your friends because they weren't there when you needed them? What did you expect? You didn't go out with them anymore, didn't accept their invitations, you kept putting them off or lamenting about things not going round. At the latest by the third time you lamented about the same subject, your friends surely didn't want to listen to you anymore. They conceive your behavior as mean, feel themselves left behind, betrayed, disappointed. Your friends can't cope with the situation. It's probably worth trying to see whether they might want to have anything to do with you again, if you start talking about other things. But if they don't, you know you tried. But honestly now, there are thousands and thousands of people around the world among which you can still find new friends, as bitter as this option may seem to you now. Make a new beginning. Grant yourself a new start, venture an attempt to break free of your little suffocating world of pain. I assure you that meeting new people will distract you, and help you appease, or even forget the pain… just like anything new captivates your attention and distracts you from pain and worries.

So, this was one of the most difficult chapters.

Yet another facet of life-quality

Let us dream a little together… Now imagine you have no obligations, you have only rights. You can dream yourself a perfect life, just the way you would like it to be. What do you think?

You have many friends and have much fun every day. Who does the housework? Who is responsible for cooking? And who for earning money to provide for such a life?

Stop! You should dream and not just set it all aside again, because you think it is your duty to take care of these things.

Or is there another alternative? You want to move, to see the world and discover new countries and civilizations. Would you choose a prescheduled flight or charter an airplane? Or would you sell everything and buy a big boat, find yourself a crew and sail across the seven seas?

Which kind of sports do you practice? How do you live? What does your environment look like? What does it smell like? What does it taste like? What does it feel like?

Dream, dream yourself a perfect life. Then compare it to your actual life. Which differences are there? Which differences can be adjusted without much difficulty? Each dream can come true when we pursue it and allow it to come into our life. It always starts with the first step, with just a little step. Start small and never stop thinking big.
Dreaming is just so important. We humans need dreams, we need a goal to pursue and achieve. Sometimes, it is good to have dreams we can never fulfill, because some dreams need to remain

unfulfilled, otherwise we risk falling into emptiness. So, when you feel you are falling short on dreams because you have gradually fulfilled them all (P.S: In this case, you are a real master of dreaming!), substitute them with new ones straightaway.

Some dreams are wishes, or as "Hans-Peter Zimmermann" once said, they are a "whim". We would have liked to fulfill it, but it is not that important after all. Real wishes nag severely on us, desperately wanting to be fulfilled. They leave us no peace, no matter how hard we try to look the other way or try to ignore them.

A brief summary:
1. Dreams are important.
2. Do whatever it takes to fulfill real dreams.
3. Never let your provision of dreams dry out, always keep at least a dream in stock.
4. Differentiate between real dreams/wishes and futile whims
5. Never feel guilty because of fulfilling your own dreams
6. Visualize dreams carefully.
7. Proceed sometimes with small steps on your way to fulfill a dream.
8. Dreams are allowed.
9. Fulfilling dreams is allowed.
10. Be crystal clear about your dreams! The clearer, the better.

But above all, attention! „Be careful what you wish for." ("It might come true."). P.S: In the meantime, I've come to know what I am talking about. Gee! If you would like to know more, just talk to me. There are many things I didn't write in here for they would go way beyond the scope of the book.

Here, an example from the television which was closely examined by researchers: Some people turn to millionaires thanks to the lottery or to a TV program. But most of them literally squander all their money within no more than a very few years. Why? Well, these people suddenly became rich, they wished for it, and there it suddenly came true. But they didn't seriously think what it means to own e.g. 1 Million Dollars. They know nothing about investment funds, they don't know what to do with so much money. The German lottery operators had thus good reasons to appoint a special, and very serious, financial adviser to support the winners. The winner deposits the money at start on short notice in a newly opened bank account, takes a trip to distance himself from day-to-day stress and to "digest" the whole matter, and finally secures the prize following on the expert's advice.

It's almost the same with our wishes. If you are in reality insufficiently (or not at all) ready to embrace your dreams and wishes, you are pretty sure to meet your waterloo.

Please, conceive your dreams carefully, think them through, ponder on what it would mean if that dream comes true, what would change in that case, like your apartment, your work, your family or your friends for instance. All these things are part of fulfilling your dream and not just the mere wish to become rich. Everything has consequences.

So, be careful with your dreams and with their realization.

Dreaming for pain patients

Let us move to the practical part for a change. As pain patient, you surely have the wish to be free of pain. I can understand this very well. Now imagine the pain would magically vanish. What would then change? What would your life be like without pain?

I am going to fantasize a little: So, you have no more pain and are happy at first. Then you start pursuing all the things you missed doing while you were ill. Some push themselves to the limit with sports, some others lunge to their career or housework, to the salary-paid job or their independent work. Most of them attempt with all their power to catch up with what passed them by.
But where's the joy? Where are the breaks and rests? What happens of self-awareness? Oops, I think I hit a raw nerve here!

Did you notice anything? As soon as you just manage to stand on your feet, you start tending to all your duties instead of tending to yourself and to the preservation of your health.

This is where it gets really exciting…

Pain Patients' "Actions" really "speaking louder than words"

You were definitely either perplexed or upset by the last few pages. You maybe even thought it was just rubbish. And yet you kept reading this far. You are a little curious after all. Well then, you are most welcome to a guided tour to more insights.

Each change goes through several stages. It starts with the realization that there is something that needs to be changed. Then it progresses into discerning the true nature of this "something"; the clearer, the exacter, the better. And then it is necessary to find a suitable solution or approach to finally implement the change.

This all sounds so simple and logical here. But still, most implementation attempts fail in the real world. As long as everything can be mind-managed, as long as it can be discussed, it is no problem. But only action is real change. Why do most people fail when it comes to this last stage?

Why, or better yet, what makes them fail to implement their ideas?

The answer is simple: Because they don't take themselves seriously enough, because they give up at the first mistake or lost battle. The alternative would be to: Stand up again whenever you fall. But you are too often ashamed of not having succeeded on your own, and here's your mindset to it: "I don't care anyway". That's it. But how can we turn the tide?

Each and every person is unique. Each person has its singularities, takes a distinct way to reach its goals and reacts differently to conversations, suggestions, advices, tips or consultations.
A preset program may suit many people, but there are many others who completely reject it, because it makes them feel too restricted.

Based on my experience, I can say with certainty: It is best to find the right mixture. In other words, you should make a mix of some perfectly suitable methods and some less suitable ones.

Top priority goes however to remaining true to yourself throughout the process of change and to keep the promises you made to yourself. Then it is going to work. Oh, I can almost see your questioning faces before me now…

First of all, set yourself a time frame and keep it, no matter what else is planned. Take your own time limits seriously. Begin with small things, such as taking lunch at 12:30 sharp a whole week long and having a good and possibly healthy meal, and taking at least half an hour lunch break. Be consistent and do this on every day of the week. Once that week has elapsed, check how you are doing. Did you manage to persevere and are you feeling good about it? Have you been true to yourself? Congratulations!
A short recapitulation: Find yourself something to stick out to for a week, and remain constant to it afterwards.
You have succeeded to make the first step. Now, proceed to the next. A few days later you realize you are slipping back into your old jog trot, giving priority to all but your plans. Your old habits are in full control. And so you learn which obstacles hinder the successful implementation of any change.

Old habits are strong, stronger than we even dare to imagine. They keep coming back without any notice. Only then when we, so to say, "catch ourselves red-handed", recidivating into old habits, when we become aware of this, we have a really good chance to make a change.

Our aimed change begins with self-observation. What do I do when…? What don't I do when…? Which measures can I undertake to avoid this…?

Here an example I experienced myself: Being independent means for example, to be liable to submit an advance turnover tax return to the fiscal authorities either every month or quarter. This means that all receipts and expenditures must be accounted for to the fiscal authorities on time and in detail. At the beginning of my career as self-employed 10 years ago, I was committed to submit this tax return to the fiscal authorities every month. And there is a submission deadline to be abided by, namely the 10th/12th of each month. I seldom sat down relaxed to collect that data at the beginning of a month. I mostly postponed this task till the last possible minute. Later on, instead of setting my tax return sheet together, I found myself filing documents, writing a letter I should have written long ago or or or… I used to find so many pretexts to dodge this unpleasant obligation, that even dusting seemed more pleasurable. As I caught myself doing so, I was taken by astonishment a brief moment at first, then I just had to laugh out loud. The curse was broken all at once. Ever since, I prepared my tax return at the beginning of every month, even if submitting it was only due at the beginning of the next quarter.

I wish and hope this example may have brought you some clarity. Learn to observe yourself. Learn as much as possible about yourself. It is essential.

As long as you don't know what makes you tick, any attempt to change will fail.

But assuming you do know yourself and whatever makes you tick very well, here comes the next stage:
What do you want to change? Think about it, all you need is small steps and a big goal to pursue. No matter how small your steps are, they will eventually lead you to success.

Imagine your big goal down to every detail; imagine what achieving it would feel like. Would your environment change? If yes, how? Will you be surrounded with new people? Who are they? Will you have a new profession? Or even a new vocation? Describe this all in detail and write it down. Only what you clearly know and understand is worthwhile.

Oh, and thanks for reminding me: What does this all have to do with pain? Most people are chronic pain patients because, deep inside their hearts, they dislike the life they lead (see Chapter IV, Case studies). There are ways to change our lives and to lead a new different life. But, what kind of life? See! This is how we get back to self-observation, or even farther back to the question about what you need to feel well.

I repeat and recapitulate...

You are tormented by this obstinately persisting pain, that doesn't want to leave you? You are suffering, aren't living your life anymore, are lonely, miserable and filled with pain... but you want this to change. Learn everything you can possibly learn about yourself and your illness. Be vigilant about the signals emitted by your body and perceive your true self. Don't let your pain drown you, not even when you are keeping a close eye on it, because that wouldn't do you any good at all, quite on the contrary. Observe... without losing yourself. Learning and understanding will find you eye to eye with your therapists.
Learning will help you understand your illness and reveal possibilities to ease, or even overcome the pain. Thus, you may accelerate your progress and improvement on your way to better pain management and – maybe - even to freedom from pain.
As soon as you discover what is beneficial for you and find the courage to put your findings into effect and to change your life, you will feel relieved. You are going to realize you are the one holding the reigns of your life...You decide what to do with it.

And here comes the hard part, namely implementation. When you put everything beneficial into effect, when you take good care of yourself, you are going to see remarkable changes.
Let yourself be inspired of whatever may be beneficial for you, choose your immediate sources of fun and enjoy them all without hesitation.

Live life to the fullest! Forge your own way of life!

Working Hand in Hand

This book is no substitute to the trustful and harmonious hand-in-hand work with your therapist, most of all with your palliative therapist. Regardless of how much change you undertake about yourself, you are going to need the support of your doctor throughout a given period of time. He is able to prescribe remedies, physical therapies, psychotherapy or acupuncture among other remedies from complementary medicine that helps stabilizing your situation. This is the fastest way to reach the quality of life you wish for.

And remember, there are millions of other people also suffering unbearable pain. Many meet in self-help groups. Recourse to your health insurance partner or to the internet, for both will provide you with reliable information on the nearest self-help group. In the following chapters of this book, you may find more about self-help groups, notably addresses to help you reach aid faster.

You surely noticed I love quotes and stories. Here's another one:

„We cannot change others, we can only change ourselves.
But by changing ourselves, we also change the world around us."
(A quote from individual psychology)

I wish you much success in your new position as your personal pain coach. Hopefully you have transformed form pain patient to pain person. This is something you will enjoy more and more in time thanks to the gigantic progress you'll achieve.

Part IV – Case Studies

An Introduction to Case Ctudies

The following case studies are only a random selection among innumerable destinies I witnessed throughout the last ten years of my life all around Germany. The names hereunder are purely fictional.

I recounted some stories in a brief description, but the names' repartition according the gender is accurate. The number of women seeking advice and support to manage pain is much higher than the corresponding number of men.

Some people learn very fast, some others very slowly, and some others never learn to do anything for their own sake, or to manage their own pain at all.

All the stories I tell you in the following are my personal observations and are not based on medical diagnosis and therapy. You will read about unique cases, which are valid only for this person in his/her personal context.

Hell with every touch

Rose is very young. She suffers upon every single physical contact with her parents since childhood. Actually, it hurts her every time anyone touches her at all. She has Fibromyalgia (FMS) and suffers all the following symptoms:
Rose retired by the age of 30, she can't pursue the profession she so dearly loves. She still lives at her parents' house, unable to find herself some free space. She dislikes herself and stays at distance from herself and her parents. She seems gentle, almost fragile one would say, but her body tells another story. She's afraid and doesn't want to live any longer. She's already been through so many therapies, but none of them helped. She is tender to touch, suffering continuously and medication doesn't seem to help. In spite of her depression, she can still smile so gently. She fears constricted places, and above all, places where humans come narrowly close to each other.
She is always tired, feels overstrained all the time and has no resilience. She can't work anymore. She gets by with promenading, driving is also possible. But the pain is always there, draining her of her strength, hindering her recovery, robbing her of the slightest chance to think afresh or to re-orient. She doesn't like this life. A life that lies ahead of her though she seems to already have it all behind her. She needs proximity and distance, but each at a time. The more proximity she seeks, the more she distances herself. She keeps visiting new doctors and having new therapies, and has a psychotherapist.

Remark: Now, it is time for her to let go of her family. It is time to gather the courage to stand up for the future, her future.

My life isn't worthwhile

John is a lively and inquisitive old man, who scored quite a few remarkable achievements in his life. He suffers infinite pains. Most of the time, he doesn't know how to survive social events or appointments because sitting down for a relatively long time torments him endlessly. Turning the chair around and sitting on it astride makes sitting a little longer endurable for him. Our talks distract him and keep him sitting a little longer too. He loves sitting at his computer, it makes him forget the pain for an hour, maybe two. He is a bright man, knows all about his illness and its treatment. He knows that titanium cages were implanted in some of his vertebrae, so that they don't crack anymore. He knows his sufferings began ever since. When the therapists hit a dead end in his treatment, they recurred to stiffening his SI, a joint which already is stabilized by strong ligaments. All he had was even more metal in his body. The dose of painkillers climbed; but he was astonishingly well-informed even on this matter. He knew all about the drugs' compositions, dosage and the minimal effectiveness values of pain patches. John is still searching for a possibility to free himself from pain…but can't find any. One day he asked me, what I would advise my pain patients who can't bear their pain anymore, whose lives are pointless. Did you just feel your heart stop beating too? It took me only a second to realize John was referring to himself. Knowing how emotionally sensitive he is, I first talked about the things that could make life worthwhile, then I discussed with him what makes life so gloomy and pointless pushing him to such despair. It turned out that John was searching for a purpose to his life. Pain and its management are in modern society a delicate subject, let alone the question on finding one's path with the age of 70. But I suddenly had an idea. Erik Blumenthal and his book about old age (starting with the 70th year of age). His book is a concrete description of the possibilities old aged people have, so that they may give sense to their lives and to others', in other words, to take part in society. John read the book and told me, on the verge of tears, that it was exactly what he needed. Almost shrinking with timidity, he told me he wanted to do something he hasn't done since youth anymore, ever since he had to learn a "reasonable profession". Sculpting. I was aghast because he was severely impaired by the pain, but he had a unique, friendly, caring and calm way to reassure me. He was so incredibly happy and excited to have another chance in life to do something he so dearly loved. I recently heard he regained a positive view of his life.

Remark: You never know how the wind will blow.

Words are my last anchor

Sally suffers pain in the chest. She fell while trying to help her brother –sitting in a wheelchair– get up stairs. She wasn't strong enough to achieve the task and while on action she slipped and fell under the wheelchair…she couldn't breathe anymore. Everyone reproached her attempt; no one cared if she got hurt, if she was alright or had been damaged by the fall. All they cared about was her brother sitting in the wheel chair. That's a few decades away.

Please mind that we are talking about a grown lady here. All she did, was suppress the pain. The doctors said, Sally there was nothing, they couldn't see anything wrong. She should just take the pills and everything should be okay. Her doctor even sent her with the newspaper clipping to the self-help group with the words: "Just go there, you are beyond therapy, no one can help you anyway. That self-help group will surely help you." P.S: This is a typical example on absolute helplessness and cluelessness of a family doctor who originally requires from himself to always find a solution. But at the point where he didn't know what to do anymore, he just sent his patient away.

This particular patient loves to talk…much. She can sometimes be very difficult. But this is her way to draw the attention she usually never gets. She always feels neglected and ignored, feels her commitment disregarded. Through wheel chair accident, she was freed from that unrewarding task. The result was a typical kind of illness that doesn't figure in any book: the need to be liked at all costs; in other words: to please everybody, except herself. She dedicated attention to everyone, took care of everyone and everything, even of cats and dogs, of the garden, the housework… everyone except herself. And because she excellently took care of everyone, no one saw how desperately in need of attention and affection she really was.

One day we had a long conversation. We talked about the need for her to tell her physiotherapist exactly where the pain is, how it spreads and that she can't breathe. Soon afterwards she called and told me she was almost free from pain. She was getting better every day. The physiotherapist had found a way to move the jolted thoracic vertebrae back in their right place.

Remark: The autonomic nervous system sees to that our breathing system functions automatically. This system is partially situated between the thoracic vertebrae. Once these vertebrae are dislodged, they can consequently also affect our breathing process. As the physiotherapist "moved" the vertebrae back into their right place, he cleared the nerve tract; the breathing mechanism could then work flawlessly again. Since the nerve tracts weren't pinched and jammed anymore, there was no more reason for them to hurt. But since they had been jammed for a very long time, she kept having pain for a while (for weeks and months) before it finally vanished.

Can't keep up anymore

Let's call it a heel spur and its consequences. Joan was in her late 50s, looking forward to an early retirement while planning a new activity, or rather seeking the dream of her life. At first, everything went well, but worries started nagging her after a while, worries about money, about whether she was going to make it just the way she dreamt it, if money would flow or if she were strong enough to reach her goal alone. These thoughts continuously kept haunting her. She was very committed, did much voluntary work, took care of her family…in other words, she put herself a 24-hour job together. Sleep, in her case, wasn't part of the plan.

In time, Joan realized she needs to set priorities, otherwise, she was running the risk of doing everything wrong and the dream she always wanted to fulfill is going to fall by the wayside.

Remark: Some people apparently can't say "NO", but what can they do about it? Such people inevitably end up on the way to illness. In this particular case, it turned out that the heel spur couldn't be treated. Now, it was up to Joan to decide what's important for her. At least, she read what Louise Hay wrote on this matter.

Hitting a dead end.

Mary suddenly began suffering somatic-sensory disorders in one of her hands, namely the hand she works with. Within no more than a few weeks, the disorder grew into extreme pain; she suffered extremely whenever anything came in touch with her hand, anything, even if it were so fine as a scarf. It was winter and she was feeling very cold.

On the phone, she told me she owns a little hotel and still does all the work herself, she said she does the beds every morning, prepares breakfast... and whatever else needs to be done in a good, personally-run hotel, although she reached an age where she didn't want to do all those things herself anymore. She sounded a little tired.

Her doctor told her she had the Sudeck's atrophy (CRPS); a degeneration of the nerves. A member of her family looked it up in the internet and found a definition and explanation of the word. But she still couldn't really understand her condition.

I managed to find a few words to explain before I sent Mary to a doctor of naturopathic and palliative medicine who masters neural therapy. This method of treatment is about Nerve Stimulation, and it really helped Mary whose pains were finally relieved.

Remark: this particular kind of disorder can only be treated and cured, if it is diagnosed and treated on a very early stage. Unfortunately, the disease is only identified very rarely because it occurs at a rate of 0.05-5% (equal to 15 000 cases in Germany per year), hitting people between their 40th and 60th year of age. It doesn't seem to affect children. The triggering factor is in most cases overseen; it can be a minor or major incident occurring at a time when the affected person is psychologically overburdened. Like fibromyalgia, Sudeck's atrophy is yet an insufficiently studied disease, which still lets us hope a possibility may be found to treat and cure even the patients whose affection was only diagnosed at a later stage.

Not forgiving me

Jenny sat down in front of me; she wanted to talk to me. No one else may be around, no one may hear what she had to say. I have had such conversations so often by now. I know what this is all about. And here it comes again, this taboo, this silent secrecy cloaking the past: The abuse of a child or a youth by a close relative. No, this is not some story about an evil stepfather or an evil stranger. When it comes to abuse, it is almost exclusively about close relatives like fathers, grandfathers, uncles or trusted neighbors.

She suffered continuously, having sometimes pain in the back, some others in the belly, sometimes it felt like having fibromyalgia. It varied. We talked about it, talked about what it felt like to keep it secret, not to find a single person to believe her story, laying the blame on childish fantasy. She underwent therapy because of this, she said. She learned to forgive her uncle. It was okay, they still get out of each other's way, she can't look him in the eyes. She can't understand how he could do that to her in the first place.

I just listened to her, took her seriously, understood, was there for her. Jenny desperately begged me not to tell anyone about this conversation. I promised her I wouldn't, and I kept my promise. I promised secrecy to every woman who ever told me a similar story, and to every man.

Only few people know of such cases, while almost no one really stops and thinks of such matters. Even men suffer abuse in their childhood.

At some point, I asked Jenny a single question: I asked her whether she had forgiven herself. I was holding her hand all through the conversation, but then I noticed she started trembling. I looked at her with questioning eyes, saw her tears and knew for sure, she had forgiven everyone but herself. She felt guilty. She felt guilty because of what happened. And she couldn't forgive herself. She knew that forgiving herself, time and time again, will make her pain fade away, and she will be free.

Remark: you surely noticed while reading that this kind of stories keep repeating themselves, over and over again. Most of the victims are women. A trauma specialist surely knows better...all I can do is understand what these people are going through, share their feelings, stand by them for a while on their path of pain. Please, if you know any victims of such abuse, tell them there are trauma-specialists. They exist, and they can help. Please, don't feel obliged to please the victims by silently knowing. Believe me, it would only make things worse. Allow the person that was a life-long burdened with this taboo, to seek specialized advice.

Pain, don't leave me all alone!

As Eve once told me about her migraine… sounding almost triumphant as she did. I was astounded to hear how she "juggled" with medications.

Her doctor prescribed her Tryptophan for emergencies only, and not at all as a long-term treatment. I was stunned when she told me, how she gets by in the meantime with other medications, how lonely she felt in her apartment.

Eve lived alone, had no friends and was very isolated. She actually drew all my attention. She spoke solely of illness and pain, had nothing else to tell. And the thought flashed through my head: she is paying an incredibly high price in exchange for a little attention.

She told me, her migraine even caused her back pain, a pain that just wouldn't yield to any treatment, same as her migraine. I went on cautiously with my questions and gradually found out she had previously suffered many diseases, most of which were pain disorders. Eve had no friends, and whenever she finds any, they run off pretty fast.

As I brought up the question of the price she was paying, she suddenly turned very reticent. Then she abruptly stood up and muttered something like "I got it already, I am not welcome here, I'll go then". Some time later, I heard that her doctor diagnosed her with medication-induced headaches.

Remark: this kind of disease counts nowadays among addictions. The drugs are in such cases no longer taken because of an illness, but because they make people feel good. The only effective treatment in such cases is abstinence, provided that the patient is carefully informed of the details first. The relapse rate is between 33 and 66% in the first five years.

Did you buy that

Once, the following conversation arose yet again in the self-help group triggered by one of the pain patients:

Susi A.
„I can't tolerate the drugs my doctor prescribed."
GL
„What kind of drugs did you get? What did your doctor say about that?"
Susi A.
„My doctor said this is completely normal."
GL
"Did you buy that?"
Susi A.
„No, of course not. This is exactly why I am not taking the medication anymore."
GL
„What did your doctor say about that?"
Susi A.
„He doesn't know."
GL
„So what are going to tell him when you visit him next time and he asks if the drugs were any help?"
Susi A.
„I am just not going to tell him at all."
GL
„Did you already do that?"
Susi A.
„Yes, last time."

GL
„Didn't he notice? He surely must have asked how you were doing?"
Susi A.
„No, he just asked me if I was alright before he gave a new prescription."
GL
„Did you have it filled already?"
Susi A.
„No."
GL
„So what are you going to do?"
Susi A.
Shrugged her shoulders and said „I'm not sure."
GL
„What's the pain doing anyway? Is it getting better or worse?"
Susi A.
„It still is same old, maybe slightly worse."
GL
„So this question remains open: Now what?"
Susi A.
„I guess I'll just have to learn to live with the pain."
GL
„Have you ever considered gathering information about yourself and talking to your doctor about the best way to provide you with medication that doesn't cause all these side effects?"
Susi A.
„Do you mean I can do that? I always thought it was wrong to argue with a doctor, or even to ask him any questions …"

Remark: There it was again, the moment you don't know whether you heard an adult talking, or a child that needs to be taken by the hand. No, I don't really despair. The age-old belief in a limitless and exclusive knowledge held by authority figures such as doctors, teachers, pharmacists and priests keeps coming to the surface again and again. It mostly brings along the fear of saying anything wrong, or rather of saying anything at all… otherwise this venerated person may not like me (anymore).

No one listens to me

When I met Matthew he had very intrusive black-blue eye circles. He looked very sad and had incessant stomachaches. After we sat a while together, he began to tell me about his pain, about his odyssey and his many doctors.

No one really helped, no one listened to him. He just keeps getting additional drug prescriptions. Since he trusts doctors and believes what they say, he just obediently takes his drugs. He finally ended up taking a row of about 40 medicaments. And his stomach ached and protested louder and louder. After we spent some time talking, his eyes turned timidly brighter until his entire face glowed bright, making even his dark eye circles disappear.

Then he told me he newly began receiving pain treatment by a special palliative doctor. This was a doctor who finally listened to him, checked up all the drugs he was taking and talked to him very frankly. Matthew said he couldn't believe he was a real junkie. With the doctor's help, he started a drug withdrawal. He was getting pretty good along in the outpatients', but he was alone. Our conversation was a slight dose of encouragement and strength for him.

Remark: unfortunately, this is not a unique case. Many doctors assured me, that about 40% of the pain patients are addicted to medication. This happens on the one hand, because most doctors don't ask what drugs are already being taken by the patient, and on the other hand, because most patients are still way too submissive to authority figures. Similarly to the way it was in the 1950s and 1960s, nothing of what the venerated Priest, Pharmacist, Teacher or doctor says may ever be questioned. This is how the lack of information would lead to a new disease. No wonder that so many pain patients still fear taking medication containing

Opioids, which are optionally given in many pain-disorder-cases, provided they are taken consistently and regularly. Taking opioid medications requires much discipline.

Summary

It is beyond doubt, that there are many other noteworthy cases. The ones here above occurred to me spontaneously and I consider them important because they frequently come about.

Throughout the years, I always asked the pain patients I met about the position they held among their siblings and about the characteristics marking their raising since childhood in general. Interestingly, most of them were either firstborns, see eldest sister or brother, or an only child. They were burdened since childhood with a critical characteristic, namely a strong sense of responsibility, responsibility to take care of others. Many questions and beliefs have their roots in our childhood. Hereunder is a short list of the most common:

- "I must always serve."
- "I may not fail."
- "I have to behave myself."
- "I must always be good."
- "I have to be perfect, otherwise I am worthless."
- "I have to prove myself through my acts and performance; otherwise no one will notice my presence."
- "It is no use, no matter what I do."
- "Right now."
- "Only I can do this."
- "I have to accomplish everything all by myself."

Does any of these statements sound familiar to you? You surely can add a few of them to the list. Are you a firstborn too?

Let us take a swift glance back at the collection of principles here above. Doesn't it reflect an extreme sense of responsibility, an adherence to the lessons learned in childhood?

What has become of these beliefs by now? Minding that I repeatedly mentioned them throughout this book, remember:

- Not being able to say NO
- Always thinking of others first
- Always serving everyone every possible way
- Always being in the service of family, friends, pets, of the garden, the housework... (the order can be changed at will)
- Not/never thinking of oneself
- Thinking of yourself immediately fills you with a sense of guilt
- Never asking for help
- Doing everything immediately all by oneself
- Never being able to hand responsibility over to a delegate
- Thinking that others can't do it anyway as good as you can, so better do it right now by myself, before having to do it all over again, etc.

No wonder that your body protested at some point in time. Not even the medications can help if you disregard your own limits. You keep getting carried away, you overstrain yourself with this impulse, with this need to make everything perfect; the apartment for instance, looks always spick and span, the garden is always perfectly trimmed, the dog's fur is so clean it shines. And what does the housewife's hair look like? It is dull and brittle. And what about her body? It is whining and wailing, aching and striking. Would you still want to „function" if you were never allowed to rest, never allowed care or recovery? Of course not! Do you know what a woman recently told me? After over 40 years of marriage, she emptied the luggage from the car all by herself while her husband was chitchatting with the neighbors on the sidewalk.

Her joints protested as she did. She also told me, she was aware of all that, but just couldn't get past the habit she acquired over the long years... getting past it was simply impossible. Besides, what would her husband say, how would he react... what if he leaves her! She could never imagine herself all alone in her old age.

Congratulations on so much self-sacrifice! Sure, her husband surely takes care of all the handcraft works in the house! Look out, this is where setting off efforts against each other starts. It is then followed by thoughts on over-responsibility, of perfection...the further development of thoughts also testifies of too much overtaken responsibility. No one stops loving the other just because he had to change a couple of habits. This partner doesn't even know you had difficulty with a particular task, in this case, emptying the luggage from the car upon your comeback from the vacation trip. He has no idea that he and his strong muscles were needed, you never told him and he is no psychic. Think of all the case studies again. Isn't it amazing how similar they suddenly seem to be?!

And now what? This is where the dilemma really begins. Let us stick to the example of emptying the car. Asking your partner for help, will kick your rollercoaster of thoughts off: If I ask him for help, he'll think I can't do it alone. But I can. He'll think I am not fit to even do the simplest things by myself. And think about yourself: Oh! That's not really so important, I can do it already! Do you hear the systematic cry of the responsibility and perfectionism echoing, pretty loud?! Again. Your partner is not going to stop loving you only because you said after 40 years of marriage: „Honey, I can't empty the car all by myself anymore. Could you please give me a hand here? We'll have plenty of time to chat later" or so. Many of the women who finally find the courage to speak out, had suppressed this urge for so long, that they just start jangling. Blustering, nagging and swearing are taboo. These are things you would really annoy your partner with. Always be friendly, don't let yourself get carried away, express yourself in a friendly, confident and determined way. In other words: set limits.

Did you notice? We are tending to the psychological facet here, exactly the same facet that always is disregarded and rejected in the course of pain therapy. That's when people barricade themselves behind the motto: "But I am not crazy". You definitely are completely normal; it's just that you are tripping yourself up, you are winding up the vicious circle of pain with the behaviors you were brought up on, because you brush your limits aside or maybe don't even know where your limits are. This is the fundament of the success, or failure, of pain therapy and management.
Breaking free of such deeply anchored patterns of behavior is the point of recurring to psychotherapy along with pain therapy. But instead, all pain patients fear of being brainwashed. And again we hit against a lack of essential information necessary to assess the disease and its actual circumstances.

Gather information, learn everything you can possibly learn about your condition, in order to get wiser, to become a better patient, to get to know yourself, to better understand your disease, to finally be able to manage your pain instead of being managed by it.

Part V – Self-help Groups

Self-help Groups

What should I expect?

- Let us take a look and ask:
- What does a self-help group do in general?
- What is the point of it? What can I learn?
- What's in it for me?
- Should I give something in return? How much does it cost?
- How can I find such a group near me?
- How do I get in contact?

Help - given and taken

Self-help groups neither grant nor receive help from the outside world. This may sound strange at first. But instead, each group member is a help to the others by helping himself. Let me explain: the members of the group help each other (mutual help); moreover, each of them demonstrates how he helped himself, thus serving as a self-help model for the others. As example: if a member manages to relax by doing given exercises, he could teach the other group members the way to perform these exercises and so they can participate in exercising at will. This is how each participant gets to decide whether the exercise is suitable for him/her or not.

You are the expert when it comes to your pain

Each person knows best about its own problems and diseases and (maybe even) the way to manage them and so, each person is responsible for the start its own expert. If you take the group

seriously, you will be surprised of the amount of knowledge gathered in it and to which extent each member can benefit from it.
In parallel, you definitely still have the possibility to refer to experts outside of the group's frame, whenever you have questions, doubts or are in need of help. Experts you should let in on your knowledge and insights.

What brings people to form a self-help group is

- The desire to better know themselves by getting to know other people
- To gather information
- Seeking the support and understanding of peers having a firsthand experience of the same problem
- Finding new friends in an environment where they feel appreciated and understood
- Supporting other members of the group
- Filling community in on problems and misunderstandings
- Participating in measures aiming to solve certain problems
- Living life in spite of hardships and diseases
- Breaking free of their isolation and loneliness

How can I find a self-help group?

That's quite simple, all you have to do is ask your health insurance company, search the internet, carefully read the newspaper, talk to your doctor or to the other patients in the waiting room or read the information displayed at the doctor's office. Some groups are dedicated to tackle respectively a precise problem, such as

- Headaches and migraine
- Fibromyalgia (FMS)
- Cancer related pain
- Interstitial Cystitis
- Rheumatism
- Back pain
- Sudeck's atrophy (CPRS)
- And many more

As soon as you find an according address, you can establish contact very easily. One phone call will be all you need to know when, where and how often the group meets, how it is structured, whether you need to join an association and so on.
Most self-help groups require no participation fees because health insurance funds financially support their work. The groups' spokespeople and leaders are volunteers who aren't paid for their work. Other groups however are structured as an association you can join. And this, in turn, means you will be required to pay membership fees.

Now to the final question: is there anything else required? Well, we already settled the financial question. Further above in the text, I explained how a self-help group in general works, how each member benefits of everyone else's experiences. It is only fair to expect you to share your story allowing others an insight to your knowledge. After all, you are granted an insight on the others' experiences too.

Throughout more than seven years of work with a self-help group, I witnessed how a committed core group of approx. 10 to 20 members came into being, while way more than 100 people occasionally took part in the group. Many came by a couple of times, collected information and left. I seldom experienced those people reveal anything about themselves at all.

Other people participated almost an entire year to the group. They gradually picked up and applied the knowledge either to partially subdue the pain, or to manage and cope with it. They were the authors of farewell messages like: "I am not going to come back anymore, I am doing well now." Goal achieved. Sometimes, the message had an additional part: "…seeing the others and their pain is depressing." That's sad because exactly these sufferers are a source of much knowledge for others. This attitude counteracts the self-help concept. Oh, and please mind: you seek the self-help group, not vice-versa.

A few words about the internet and its utilization

Nowadays, there is a reference to any information broadcasted on television, in the radio, in newspapers or books on the internet and even of lectures and seminars.
Everyone is now somehow on the internet. Google, one of the greatest internet search-engines, just reported having 1 Billion (that is a 1 followed by 12 (twelve) zeroes: 1,000,000,000,000) different websites, still growing. Even Google's staff was astonished by this record. This means there is an unimaginable amount of information available online. But this doesn't necessarily have to mean, that all the info is useful, interesting or correct.

So where is the difference between a „good" and a „bad" information?

At first sight, nothing. Only after scrutiny and extended reading you manage, in time and thanks to much accumulated knowledge and expertise, to discern which sites you should better not waste your time reading. I would like to elucidate anyhow.

Let us begin with the „bad" information:
It is mostly presented as the only and irrevocable truth, repudiating all other opinions, illustrations or conceptions. It insists on being the only information that is right and useful. It is superficial and only seldom bears up scrutiny. Often, it has no references or links. Many text pages offer only incomplete information, which is not always deliberately decided by its author whose writings are

conditioned by his biased knowledge. Many sites are overburdened with advertisements, but this is not necessarily a sign of meager quality. Yet, you should be skeptical: plenty of such websites just represent advertisement masked as information.

„Good" information always is comprehensive and detailed, rarely leaving any questions unanswered. It is well-founded and corroborated with further sources of information. But please don't mistake technical terms with bad information. Ideally, the information should be understood without the need to refer to a dictionary, which is not always the case. You should have the courage to read this kind of information as well. Almost every technical term can be looked up on Wikipedia by now. And since it has recently tightened its quality standards, you can look up anything on a corresponding wiki website.

For valuable and relevant information, it is always worthwhile to refer to the websites of related organizations or institutions. They don't claim to be wisdom's exclusive owners, quite on the contrary, they are trying their best to present all available information the best possible way. Please see the list of internet-links at the end of the book, there you will find much valuable information.

International Links

American Holistic Health Association
www.ahha.org

American Chronic Pain Association
www.theacpa.org

National Pain Foundation (Ambassador-Program)
www.painconnection.org

American Academy of Pain Medicine
www.painmed.org

American Pain Foundation
www.painfoundation.org

American Pain Society
www.americanpainsociety.org

Change Pain ®
www.pain-workshop.com

PAIN Association Scotland
www.painassociation.org

The Bone and Joint Decade – Global Alliance for Musculo-skeletal Health
www.boneandjointdecade.org

Stories for Encouragement and Relaxation

Washing away the pain

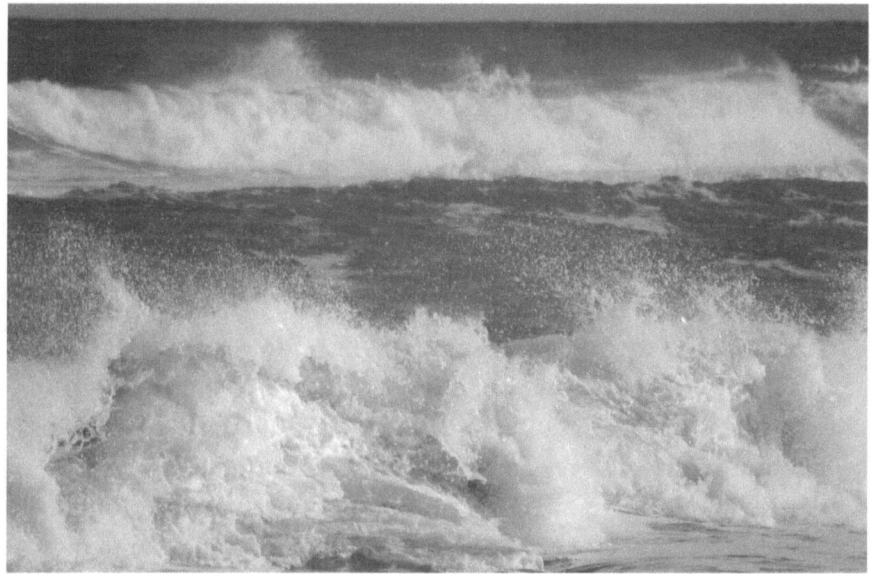

The Wave, © Heike Riesterer

This exercise is a visualization in which you imagine raindrops washing away your pain. (...) Sit in a balanced posture - remember not to slouch. (If you lie down, don't fall asleep!)

1. Close your eyes and imagine that you are walking in your favourite park. Try to recall it in as much detail as possible. Use all your senses - conjure up smells and sounds as well as sights.
2. As you visualize yourself walking, imagine that your pain is rising to the surface of your body, transforming itself into pleasant, tingling sensations all over your skin. Your pain has migrated here. This is the first step in obtaining some relief.
3. It begins to rain - a few drops at first, becoming a shower. You don't mind the rain: it is warm, gentle and refreshing. After about a minute it subsides and then stops. Lift your arms and think about how they feel - the rain has „washed away" the prickling sensation on your skin. Be aware of your face - no more tingling there either. You have been cleansed of the worst of your pain: what remains is definitely diminished.
4. You feel jubilant and „light". Stay in your park for as long as you like. When you come out of your meditation, open your eyes and be happy that you still feel light and free. Smile. Carry this feeling of lightness with you for as long you can.

Quoted from: Conquer Pain: The natural way © Leon Chaitow exercise 9, page 69
(printed with the kind permission of Leon Chaitow)

The fable of the deaf frog... or Lesson 1

Once a climbing competition was arranged by tiny frogs. The goal was to reach the top of a very high tower. A big crowd of frogs had gathered around the tower to see the race and cheer on the contestants.

The race began.

No one in the crowd really believed the tiny frogs would ever reach the top of the tower, so they shouted phrases like: "What a pity! They will never make it, not in a million years!"

The tiny frogs began collapsing, one by one, except for one frog that continued to climb higher and higher. And the crowd continued to yell: "...pity! No one will make it!..." so the frogs gave up and admitted defeat, except for the one stubborn frog that went on climbing.

At the end, all the other had given up but he alone, and with enormous efforts, reached the top of the tower. Everyone else wanted to know how he managed such a great feat.

So one of the quitters approached him to ask him how he had done it and discovered that the winner was...deaf!

Never listen to people who have the bad habit of being negative and pessimistic...for they steal the deepest aspirations of your heart!

Always think of the power of the words you hear and read; and endeavor to deafen your ears to negativity Be always POSITIVE!

In a nut shell:
Choose to be deaf towards everyone who tells you that you can't fulfill your dreams.

Always remember: YOU can make it too!

© *unknown*

Part VI – Appendix

Questionnaire about pain

You receive a form like this from your doctor ahead of the initial examination, so that he may have a general picture about your disease. It contains questions about where is your pain located, when is the pain the most intense etc.

Hereunder you will see abstracts of a German one, reprinted with the kind permission of the German Pain Association "Gesellschaft für Schmerztherapie e.V.", Oberursel.

Hatten Sie in den vergangenen vier Wochen **aufgrund seelischer Probleme** irgendwelche Schwierigkeiten bei der Arbeit oder anderen alltäglichen Tätigkeiten im Beruf bzw. zu Hause (z.B. weil Sie sich niedergeschlagen oder ängstlich fühlten)?

	ja	nein
Ich habe weniger geschafft, als ich wollte.	O	O
Ich konnte nicht so sorgfältig wie üblich arbeiten.	O	O

Inwieweit haben die Schmerzen Sie in den vergangenen vier Wochen **bei der Ausübung Ihrer Alltagstätigkeiten zu Hause und im Beruf behindert**?

überhaupt nicht	ein bisschen	mäßig	ziemlich	sehr
O	O	O	O	O

In diesen Fragen geht es darum, wie Sie sich fühlen und wie es Ihnen in den **vergangenen vier Wochen** gegangen ist (bitte kreuzen Sie in jeder Zeile den Begriff an, der Ihrem Befinden am ehesten entspricht). Wie oft waren Sie in den **vergangenen vier Wochen** ...

	immer	meistens	ziemlich	manchmal	selten	nie
... ruhig und gelassen	O	O	O	O	O	O
... voller Energie	O	O	O	O	O	O
... entmutigt und traurig	O	O	O	O	O	O

Wie häufig haben Ihre körperliche Gesundheit oder seelischen Probleme in den vergangenen vier Wochen Ihre **Kontakte zu anderen Menschen** (Besuche bei Freunden, Bekannten, usw.) beeinträchtigt?

immer	meistens	manchmal	selten	nie
O	O	O	O	O

M.Bullinger & I.Kirchberger; SF-12; © Hogrefe-Verlag

4.) **Seit wann** bestehen Ihre Schmerzen?
- ○ weniger als 1 Monat
- ○ ½ bis 1 Jahr
- ○ 2 bis 5 Jahre
- ○ 1 Monat bis ½ Jahr
- ○ 1 bis 2 Jahre
- ○ mehr als 5 Jahre

Können Sie ein **genaues Datum** angeben? ⎿__⏌ ⎿__⏌ ⎿__⏌
(Tag) (Monat) (Jahr)

5.) Haben Sie **ein einziges Schmerzbild** oder können Sie **mehrere verschiedene Schmerzbilder** (z.B. Kreuz- und Knieschmerzen; verschiedene Kopf- und Gesichtsschmerzen) voneinander unterscheiden?
- ○ ein einziges Schmerzbild
- ○ zwei Schmerzbilder
- ○ mehrere Schmerzbilder

6.) Welche der Aussagen trifft auf Ihre **Schmerzen** in den letzten 4 Wochen am besten zu?
(Bitte nur eine Angabe machen!)

— Dauerschmerzen — | — Schmerzattacken —

- ○ ... mit leichten Schwankungen
- ○ ... mit starken Schwankungen
- ○ ... dazwischen schmerzfrei
- ○ ... auch dazwischen Schmerzen

Wenn Sie unter Schmerzattacken leiden, ...

... **wie lange** dauert dann durchschnittlich eine Schmerzattacke?
- ○ Sekunden/ Minuten
- ○ Stunden
- ○ bis zu drei Tage
- ○ länger als drei Tage

... **wie oft** treten Ihre Schmerzattacken zur Zeit auf? (Mehrfachangaben sind möglich)
- ○ mehrfach täglich
- ○ einmal täglich
- ○ mehrfach wöchentlich
- ○ einmal wöchentlich
- ○ mehrfach monatlich
- ○ einmal monatlich
- ○ seltener, wie oft pro Jahr: _____

7.) **Seit wann** bestehen Ihre Hauptschmerzen in ihrer **heutigen Stärke und Ausprägung**?
- ○ von Beginn an
- ○ seit ⎿__⏌ Wochen bzw. ⎿__⏌ Monaten bzw. ⎿__⏌ Jahren

8.) Geben Sie im Folgenden die **Stärke Ihrer jeweiligen Schmerzen** an. Kreuzen Sie **auf den unten aufgeführten Linien** an, wie stark Sie Ihre Schmerzen (auch unter Ihrer üblichen Medikation) empfinden. Die Zahlen können Ihnen bei der Einteilung helfen: Ein Wert von 0 bedeutet, Sie haben keine Schmerzen, ein Wert von 10 bedeutet, Sie leiden unter Schmerzen, wie sie für Sie nicht stärker vorstellbar sind. Die Zahlen dazwischen geben Abstufungen der Schmerzstärke an.

Pain scale and journal

Here, you can see two pages of the official pain journal of the DGSS, which your doctor should hand out to you. You should note in it, the time and severity of the pain you suffered on each day, the circumstances etc. The scale of pain is represented in this journal with numbers between 0 and 10. 0 indicates the absence of pain and 10 indicates the maximum pain imaginable.

The printouts can be found in different colors or layouts, but they all follow the same principle and are all for free. Some of them are even illustrated with faces, each with a grimace representing the respective pain scale, see below.

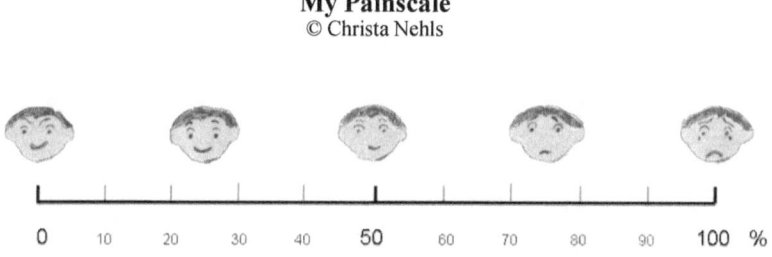

My Painscale
© Christa Nehls

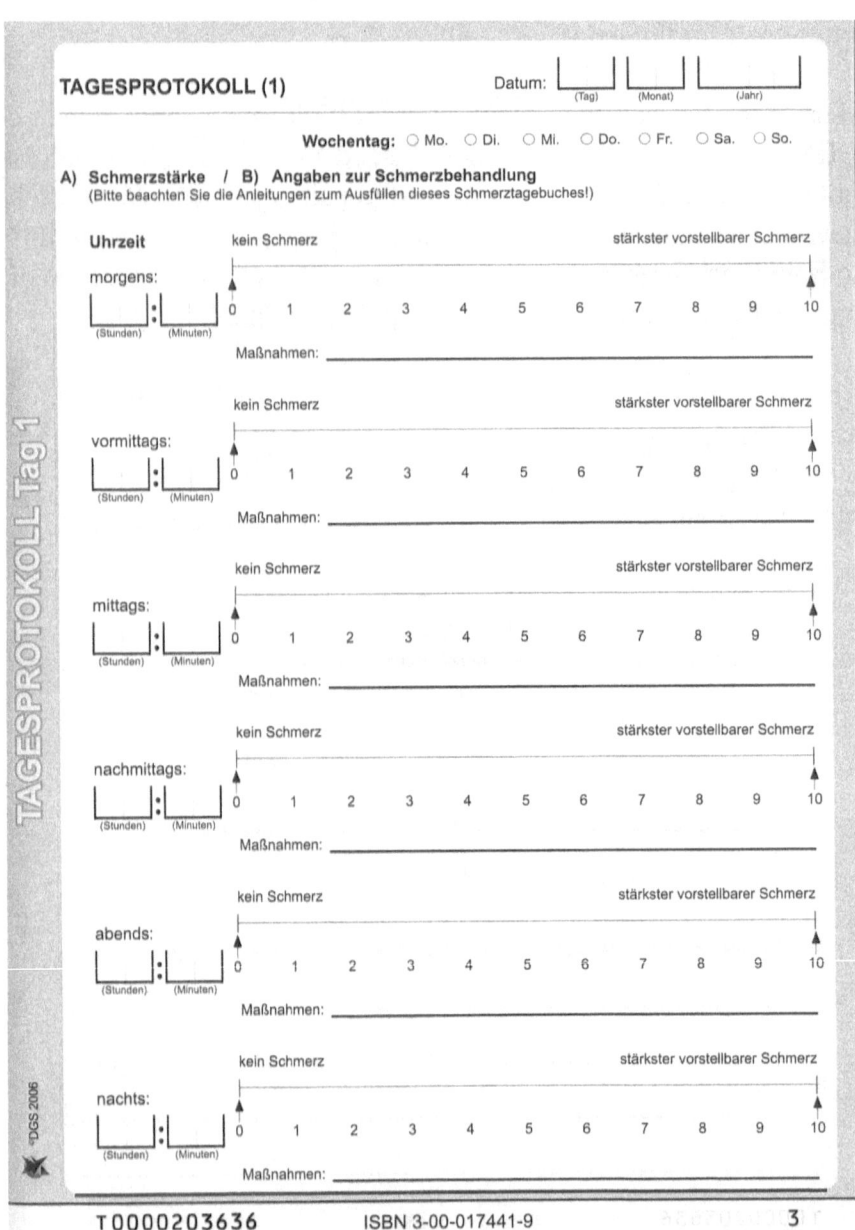

Erträglichkeit/ individuelles Behandlungsziel

Bei welcher **Schmerzstärke** wären die Schmerzen für Sie **erträglich**?

kein Schmerz — stärkster vorstellbarer Schmerz

0 1 2 3 4 5 6 7 8 9 10

C) Tagesablauf (am Abend auszufüllen)

1. Wie war Ihr **allgemeines Wohlbefinden**? Ordnen Sie Ihrem Befinden eine Position auf der Linie zu, wobei „-100" einem sehr schlechten Befinden und „+100" einem sehr guten Befinden entspicht. Machen Sie eine Markierung an der Stelle, die Ihrem Befinden entspricht.

sehr schlecht −100   0   sehr gut +100

2. War Ihre nächtliche **Schlafdauer**: ○ ausreichend   ○ nicht ausreichend

3. Hatten Sie **Dauerschmerzen**? ○ nein   ○ ja

4. Wurden Sie durch Ihre Schmerzen **in Ihren Tätigkeiten und Bedürfnissen eingeschränkt**?
   ○ nein   ○ ein wenig   ○ deutlich   ○ stark   ○ fast völlig

5. Haben die Schmerzen Ihre **Stimmung beeinträchtigt**?
   ○ nein   ○ ein wenig   ○ deutlich   ○ stark   ○ sehr stark

6. Hatten Sie das Gefühl, die **Schmerzen lindernd beeinflussen** zu können?
   ○ nein   ○ ein wenig   ○ deutlich   ○ stark   ○ sehr stark

7. Hatten Sie **sonstige Beschwerden**? (Mehrfachnennungen möglich)

   ○ keine   ○ Müdigkeit   ○ Niedergeschlagenheit
   ○ Übelkeit   ○ Appetitlosigkeit   ○ Lustlosigkeit
   ○ Magenbeschwerden   ○ Schlafstörungen   ○ Schwindel
   ○ Konzentrationsstörung   ○ Schwitzen   ○ Verstopfung

   ○ andere: _____

   © G. Müller-Schwefe, H. Seemann, D. Jungck, T. Flöter

8. Besondere schmerzbezogene Ereignisse, Ergänzungen und andere Bemerkungen:

   _____
   _____
   _____
   _____
   _____

T0000203636   ISBN 3-00-017441-9

© DGS 2006

Closing Word

This is the end of this book. Did you wish for more? Then start reading it all over again.

Did you know that the journey can be very exciting? If you work on it intensively, you will discover that a smooth transition only happens in a perfect world.

Finally you'll discover you took this whole process too lightly, supposing that brushing it over would do. Well, then you noticed that the chapter titles grew smaller, in the contrary to the efforts you must invest on yourself. So much for the "brush it over" theory!

Over the last years, I met many people – not to mention myself – who freed themselves from the vicious circle of pain thanks to this process. I didn't really know most of them; their success relied on them, on listening to their bodies and souls and finding out their real needs. This was proof enough for me to see how evident the process really is; so evident that it was issued in written in Scotland and published among the local self-help groups.

Do you still remember the preface: "I beg your pardon, I never promised you a rose garden", there's got to be a little rain sometime on the hard path from being a suffering, dependent pain patient to a lively, independent pain person. "From pain patient to pain person", what a wonderful wordplay! once upon a time created by the Scottish Pain Association.

There is still so much to say, let's call it a day, meet you in the next book!

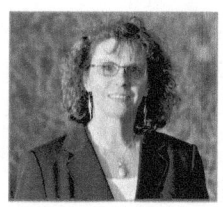

Contact:

Christa Nehls

Coach & Trainer
for Specialists and Executives
Author & Consultant

Krappmühlstraße 17
D-68165 Mannheim

Phone: +49-621 44069100
Mobile: +49-170 3023302
menschin@menschin.com
www.menschin.com

www.ingramcontent.com/pod-product-compliance
Lightning Source LLC
Chambersburg PA
CBHW020053170426
43199CB00009B/269